Helper to Fitness Coach

An epic journey of a girl who transformed her own life and others along the way

Amanda Nav

Helper to Fitness Coach

Copyright © 2021 Amanda Nav

All Rights Reserved.

The information contained in this book is based on the life experiences and opinions perceived and expressed by the author.

Published, distributed, and printed in the United States of America by Rose Gold Publishing, LLC.

ISBN: 978-1-952070-30-3

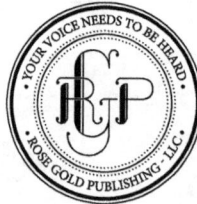

www.RoseGoldPublishingLLC.com

Amanda is an extraordinary woman, she keeps chasing her dreams until they become her reality, and the fire inside her soul, is unstoppable to light up her fellow woman to step up and find their purpose and be a better person.

-Sylvia Nathan

I have high respect for Amanda because she gives so much value to her viewers, and students. I admire her determination and perseverance she really walks the talk.

-Ramba Olido

To become an influence, you have to be a good content creator.

Winalyn Navarro

She don't just imagine and wishing things but she took action immediately. As Amanda said, your dream is bigger than your excuses. Her heart is pure.

-Lu Alivio

She makes things possible.

-Janice Gatchalian

I've seen Amanda how she work hard toward her life vision while working as a HELPER. She showed her mistakes and she's authentic showing up to the world until she gets what she wanted in life. After listening to her very first presentation about her upcoming company, all I wanted now is to be with her.

-Aila Ramirez

Foreword

By Swarnajeet Mukherjee

Another beautiful soul was born with many dreams in her mind, but circumstances shackled and shattered her dreams. **She was raped, abused, and diagnosed with cancer**.

Despite all the challenges, she never gave up. She joined the domestic helping services to keep her family fed, which would allow her to survive each day. She sacrificed everything for others until she realized her real purpose and mission in life – *Living for Others.* Even though the world was not easy on her, she continued to dream. A dream that kept her going.

One of her dreams was to meet Oprah Winfrey. So, she decided to write a letter pouring her heart out, but that letter never reached Oprah. She tried and tried, but nothing happened. None of this would break her. She became more robust. She never gave up on any of her dreams because she was not born to surrender; she was born to win, thrive, and fulfill a purpose that will impact millions of underprivileged women worldwide. A soul, a body, energy, and a never-ending fire that no storm can scare, no obstacle can stop, and no disbelieve can break. She is no other than Amanda, and this book is her story.

Read with love, care, and compassion, and you will find Amanda in your own life. Amanda is not just a name; it is a movement, a belief, and a ray of hope.

Dedication

This book is dedicated to all those who are suffering and struggling in their life worldwide. Allow me to be your fuel for a long and challenging journey. In the end, it is a rewarding journey. Allow me to be your sister and walk by your side. You will find many secrets about how you can discover your hidden talents, as I have done. You will learn how to overcome fear while working as a helper. I'm glad you that you chose to pick this up and invest your time in reading it. Thank you and enjoy the journey.

I intend to serve the world.

My dream is to save the world.

Acknowledgments

It would help if you learned to be grateful for somethings in life. Nobody can achieve great things in life without the right support, guidance, help, and inspiration. I am truly thankful for many things in my life that have made me who I am today. I have picked a handful of people who hold a special place in my life, but there are countless others, too, and I am grateful for them. So even if you are not mentioned here, know that I appreciate you.

To my employer, Esther, and her family: I want to take this opportunity to thank my employer, Esther, so much for taking care of me and treating me as one of her family members. I am grateful for everything. You made me feel at home from the very beginning. I have had the opportunity to serve you for five years now, and I can feel even a greater sense of belonging. You and your family became the fuel to my fire. Just what I needed. You fed me well and helped me create my own space for my personal development, especially for my fitness activities. I experienced life as I never had before. Esther, you showered me to care when I was feeling ill; you took me to the doctor when you could have focused on your own needs. I will never forget your kindness as now it is my mission to pay it forward and let other people feel as much love as you have given me. I hope to make you proud of all the contributions and support you have given me.

To Swarnajeet Mukherjee: You became my first Mentor and helped me when I was lost. You took me under your wings. Thank you so much for all the great help and incredible mentorship. You let me try new things and helped me narrow down on my passion and purpose. With your help, my hidden talent slowly but steadily became visible. You let me implement unconventional things and encouraged me to try new things that made me uncomfortable. Mentor, you helped me bring out my inner greatness. I applied everything you taught me, and it all works! You are my hero and thank you for believing in me. You are the reason why I started writing my story. This approach helped me get over my vulnerabilities and empowered me to become the best version. I can accept and embrace myself for who I am. I can't thank you enough for editing and proofreading my book. You helped me to express my emotions in the best way possible. It's now my turn to tell the world about the greatness in you as a mentor.

To my sister, Arlene, and her husband, Arnel: I will be grateful to both of you forever. I am blessed to have you as my sister as you helped me build my confidence to write this story and reach out to the publishing industry to have this story told far and wide. I owe you for this!

To Petra Tahanevo: Thank you so much for introducing me to Mentor Swarnajeet. I appreciate your noticing my videos on my Facebook. My skills are no longer invisible. I will treasure you and value you as my friend forever.

To Oprah Winfrey: You have always inspired me. Your life story made me realize that even a person with a tragic story like mine can live their dreams. That is why I am dedicating this book to you. You caught my attention when I was working as a helper in Saudi Arabia in 2008. I wasn't allowed to watch television then, but I happened to see you once while my employer's baby was with me and the parents were attending a party. They left their television on by accident, and I saw you for the first time. I knew then that the Universe was giving me a sign. I felt a divine calling to be the instrument of inspiration and power to all women worldwide. My heart belongs to the helper community worldwide, all because of your charismatic presence and inspiration.

To Vishen Lakhiani, I want to thank you for posting your six-phase meditation on YouTube. By listening to this repeatedly, I found great clarity on how to visualize my ambitions. Every day, I would implement the six-phase meditation twice a day, and it brought my subconscious mind into excellent condition. I became talented and smart. I was able to write my story without hiding anything anymore. I got to reassure the Universe has a plan for me. I know it is not an accident that I tuned in to your powerful meditation. I will be forever grateful to you.

To Sir John Westnedge, I will be forever grateful to you for taking a professional video and pictures every time I was teaching high-intensity workout during my off days. Without you, I won't be able to add great photos to my book. I remember the days I was dreaming of having high-quality videos and photos to have something to upload on my Facebook timeline so I can attract more fellow helpers and others to join my HIIT class for me to help others. I used to upload a low-quality video that always has a dark background and not presentable. Then I applied a video filming meditation exercise, surrendered everything to the higher power, and I was surprised- suddenly Sir John became my friend on Facebook.

Most of my request was always granted through meditation. Thank you so much for your effort and kindness, and also I am grateful for providing us free mentorship. You are one of a kind. The two things I have had learned from you were. If you want to be successful, it's ok to make mistakes. You will discover who you are as a person and keep providing free service, then blessings follow.

To my family, and especially my Mom: Thank you for your patience and for taking care of my children. At times, money was short, but you could feed my kids and care for them. I have a dream, a dream to rise from poverty and impact millions of lives suffering. I don't want people to suffer as I did, and that's why I am writing this book because I want the best for all of you. Thank you for all your kindness and support.

I am grateful to those who supported and prayed for me in accomplishing this project for the Christian community. Thank you so much. I want to thank the city of foreign domestic helpers who showed me generous support in achieving this project.

To my best friend, Grace: Without you, I wouldn't have the incredible photos to put on my book cover. I am grateful for all the nice pictures you have taken. You see me with so much love and kindness, and I am very grateful.

To my friend, Lympia: Thank you for encouraging me when I was about to give up ... and that is the perfect word ... you filled me with courage. You are the only person who patiently listened to me when I was down. We talked endlessly about my dream. You supported me even though you knew it would be hard to achieve. Thank you for having faith in my potential.

To the Naysayers: I am also highly grateful to those who doubted me and didn't believe in me. That disbelieving act made me work 100X harder to break free from my shackles and achieve things that others thought were not possible. In the end, everything happens for a reason.

I am grateful to the Universe for having my back.
Now it is my turn to serve the world.

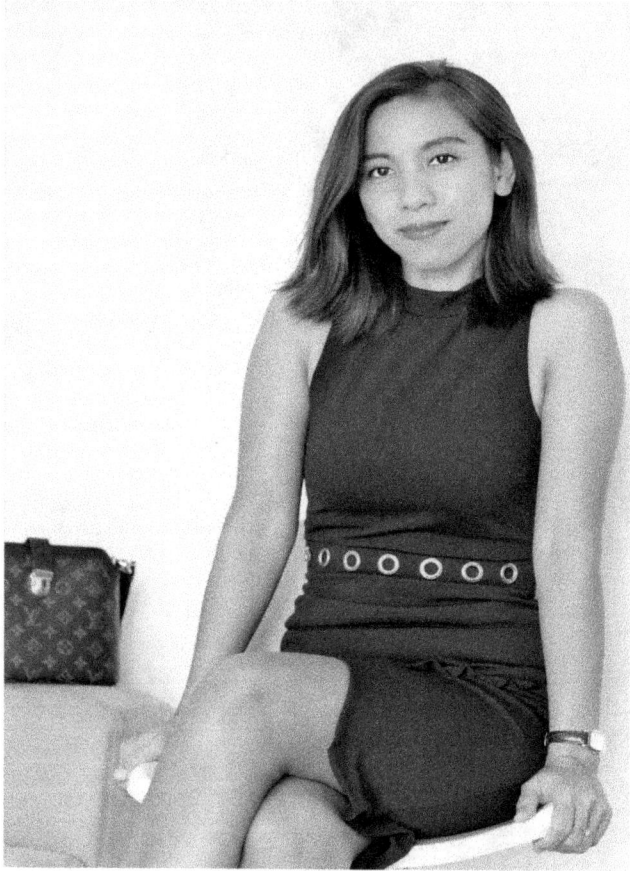

Amanda Nav

Highlights

- She was raped at age 9. Only two years ago, in 2018, she finally healed her inner soul and let go of her past.
- She has worked as a helper for over 24 years since she was 13 years old.
- She became an entrepreneur while working as a helper, and she entered a networking business.
- She has incredible stories to tell to the world. Everyone who has heard them has been inspired and often encouraged to tears. Readers have saluted her for being independent. She believes people will get tremendous value from her story.
- She hired a world-renowned life and business coach when she couldn't figure out what she wanted in life.
- She wants to make a difference in the whole world.
- She is fascinated with the idea of meeting Oprah Winfrey.
- Her dream is to be part of Lisa Nichol's tribe and learn about Lisa's speaking strategies.

- She has written her own story from childhood through today.
- She overcame many chronic diseases from her toxic childhood environment.
- She applied the principles she learned in the book "Think and Grow Rich." She was surprised at how everything unfolded, as the book said. She believes all of her dreams are possible and achievable.
- She learned to create space for her personal growth. Her job didn't stop her from soaring high, and now she's enjoying sharing her talents.
- She has applied daily meditation. Mentorship taught her a tremendous lesson and changed everything.
- She looks forward to advising and bringing value to the younger generation.
- She embraces fitness and has achieved her desired physique.
- She has found her purpose through the challenging journey of being a helper.
- She plans to become a public speaker and a transformational coach.
- She sees all her dreams unfolding within the next three years, although she would be happy to have them come true sooner.

- Her heart belongs to the helpers, employees, and laborers. She wants her voice to be heard by employers, CEOs, and founders so they can discover her hidden talent.
- Above all, her dreams is to build a school for humanity focuses on self-development and bring all the world-class teacher and experts.

Amanda's social platforms

LinkedIn:http://linkedin.com/in/amanda-nav-92099b17a

Instagram: fitness_amanda_nav_

Facebook: https://www.facebook.com/iDiana82

YouTube Channel:

https://youtube.com/channel/UCIFfm86uDbDLiCHdLZWz6
LA

Table of Contents

Introduction

Hi everyone, I'm Amanda Navarro, the author of this book. Before I tell you my story, I would like to thank you for giving me this opportunity to share my life story with you. I have wanted to share my life with the whole world for quite some time because I know my information is unique. I believe many people can relate to my experiences, and that's why I told myself that these experiences must be shared to impact others. The problem was that I didn't have someone to turn to for help and advice.

One day, a friend recommended that I find a talented mentor in many different areas. This Mentor was the one who discovered my skills. He said that I have potential, and I believed him. He told me that I have a story to share with the world. I am forever grateful to my Mentor.

Amanda's Mission and Vision

As you can see, Amanda is obsessed with fitness and healthy living. She wants to make everyone fit and healthy. The following is her mission in life:

- To create a massive community of men and women who can say, "I'm in the best shape of my life right now at this very moment. I feel amazing, and I'm ready for anything."
- To empower and inspire individuals to achieve and maintain their best quality of life by providing the best training and going beyond their expectations.
- To create an environment that encourages a healthy and positive change in everyone.
- To make fitness viral, believing fitness and a healthy lifestyle can lead to happiness.
- To create an environment where everyone can have a better quality of life.

Fitness was Amanda's first calling from the Universe. While she was training to be a fitness coach and acquiring different skill sets, she discovered another interesting calling from the Universe. You will find out more in the upcoming chapters.

Chapter 1: Background

I grew up in a rural part of the Philippines on a hillside with my brothers, sisters, and parents. It was tranquil; our neighbors were far from each other. We had no electricity, and we were very far from the city. At the age of eight, I started to experience many ups and downs in life - pains, struggles, and difficulties. My family and I worked under the hot sun together all day to earn enough to survive. Before we went to bed, my mom told us a story about her suffering when she was 24 years old. She was diagnosed with a tumor in her head and told it was stage 2 cancer. She was admitted to a public hospital, where she stayed for more than three months.

My mom underwent chemotherapy. They cut her hair. Due to the cobalt's effect, her neck was all black. My mom suffered lots of difficulties, and both of my parents struggled with finances during that period. During her three months in the hospital, the people there took such good care of her and never stopped offering healing prayer every single day.

One day, the doctor decided to operate on the tumor in my mom's head since chemotherapy wasn't working. My mom's eyesight had also been affected by cancer, so that she couldn't see clearly. Both of my parents agreed to the surgery since it seemed like the last resort. My mom prepared herself for the operation.

The day that the doctor scheduled her surgery, he and his assistants surrounded my mom's bed. Everything was already set up. Then suddenly, my mom begged the doctor to redo the scan since she felt good, fantastic, and striking that day. The doctor smiled and said to my mom, today is the day of your surgery, and again, my mom begged the doctor. The doctor finally agreed. He said, "Okay, let me scan again."

The x-ray showed that the tumor had disappeared. Everyone was in awe and happy. It was nothing but the blessings of God. She was very grateful to all the people who supported her and prayed nonstop for her healing. It's a fantastic story. There is much more story to tell, but the rest, they say, is history.

After a few months, my mom got pregnant, and I was born.

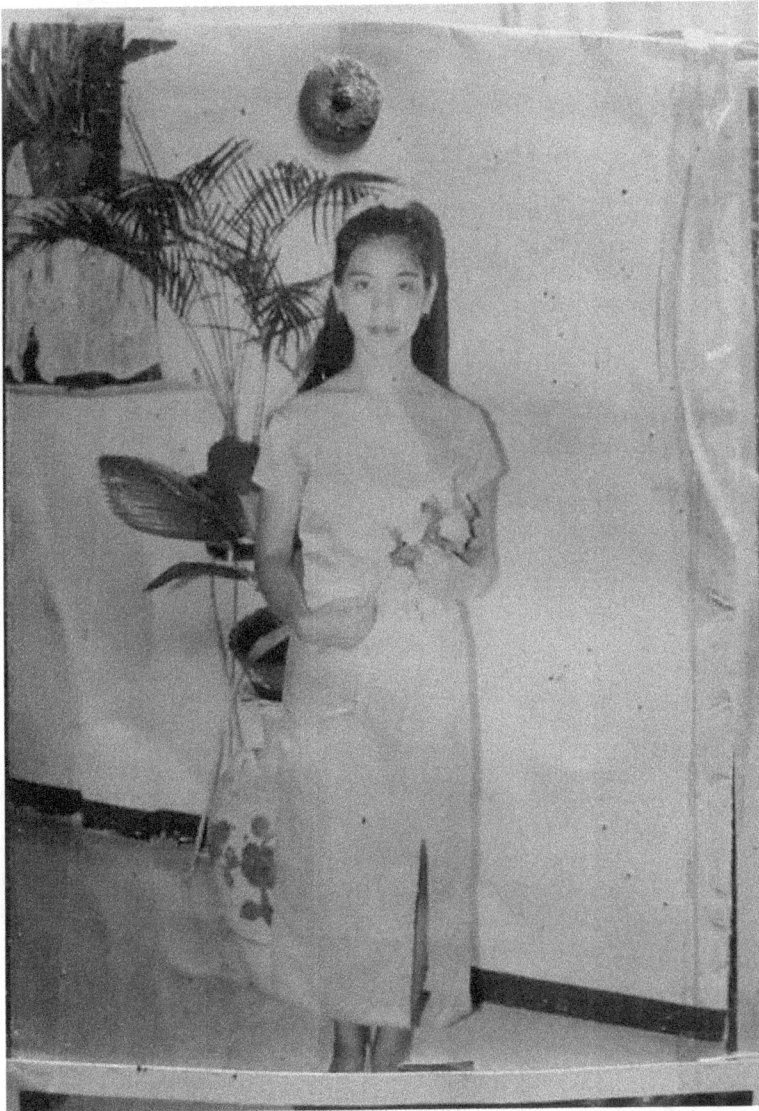

I didn't allow my childhood to shape my destiny

Chapter 2:
Own Health Challenges

When I was 18 years old, I was diagnosed with cancer. Before that, I was working as a helper for one of the wealthiest families in our town. I had just freshly graduated from Secondary School at that time, and I applied as a helper. When I got up in the morning, I felt something very unusual happen to my body. I felt a pain in my neck that morning. When I touched it, there was a big lump on the left side of my neck. It was hard and big. I went to the mirror, and there I saw this big lump. It was very noticeable. I was nervous.

I waited for my employer to get up to tell her about the lump. Sadly, this employer didn't care much about me. She let me pack my things, and I went back home. I told my mom what happened. The next day, we went to the hospital. The doctor gave me a referral to go to the Manila City Hospital, where they could scan and do a biopsy because it might be cancer. The doctor didn't tell me his opinion that it might be cancer. My Mom and I went back home, laughing together while we walked instead of dwelling on it. We were laughing because we didn't know where to get cash to pay for this journey.

A few weeks later, I went to Manila by myself. It took me 7 hours to travel by bus. I met the doctor. The lump had filled with pus. He used a syringe to take out the puss for the biopsy. The doctor said to come back after two days, which made me nervous. What was this thing growing on my neck?

My skin was dry, and I looked very unhealthy. I stayed with our relatives 3 hours away from the clinic. To pay for staying in their home, I woke up early, washed their clothes, and did all the household chores. I am thankful to this family because, even though I worked hard, I saved money.

When I returned for the results, the doctor told me that the syringe was missing. MISSING. How could that be?

So, he did another biopsy. I saw the two syringes he filled with pus. I was curious and asked the doctor, "Why is there so much pus inside the lump? Is it dangerous? Am I going to get well?" The doctor replied, "I will let you know once I find out the results. For now, relax and don't panic." The doctor was not aware that I was staying far away from the city and that this was another massive challenge. He asked me to come back again after two days. I left the clinic with a sudden sadness, worry, and nervousness. After two days, I went back to the clinic and quickly asked for the results. The doctor said, "It is cancer. It needs surgery as soon as possible so that it won't spread to some other part of your body." He also added that I should have someone accompany me.

I begged the doctor and told him we were poor. We couldn't afford the surgery. He then prescribed one month's medication and told me to come back for another check-up. He said it was essential to see him personally. I left the clinic with heavy sadness and teary eyes. I went back home to my mother. While I was on the long bus ride home, I wondered where I could get money to buy the medicine.

When I got home, I told my mom the whole story because she was worried about me. I sat in a corner almost every day and cried. I was so disappointed in my life. My mom was busy trying to find people who could help us buy medicine. She went to our local municipality, where she could ask for help. Some people gave her cash, and she purchased my medication. Few people talked about my sickness; I was embarrassed to face people. Some of my friends and family visited me and tried to comfort me.

One day, while I was listening to a radio program, everything changed. The broadcaster's topic was all about "How To Cure Cancer Naturally Without Surgery." The announcer shared tips about the benefits of potatoes and carrots for cancer patients. Eat boiled potatoes and carrots for at least six months, and you will be amazed by the results. I followed what she said.

I took some medication, but I didn't complete what the doctor prescribed since we didn't have enough money to buy it. I also ate sweet potatoes. When the doctor asked me to come back for the next appointment, I didn't go because we didn't have money again. I continued to consume carrots, potatoes, and sweet potatoes.

One of our relatives took me to spiritual healing. They used coconut sticks to burn my neck. It was painful, but they said you must believe or you won't be healed. I went back home with lots of burns on my neck. Everyone was staring at me and asked what had happened. I kept quiet and didn't respond to their questions. Gradually, the lump disappeared and faded from my thoughts. I was healed.

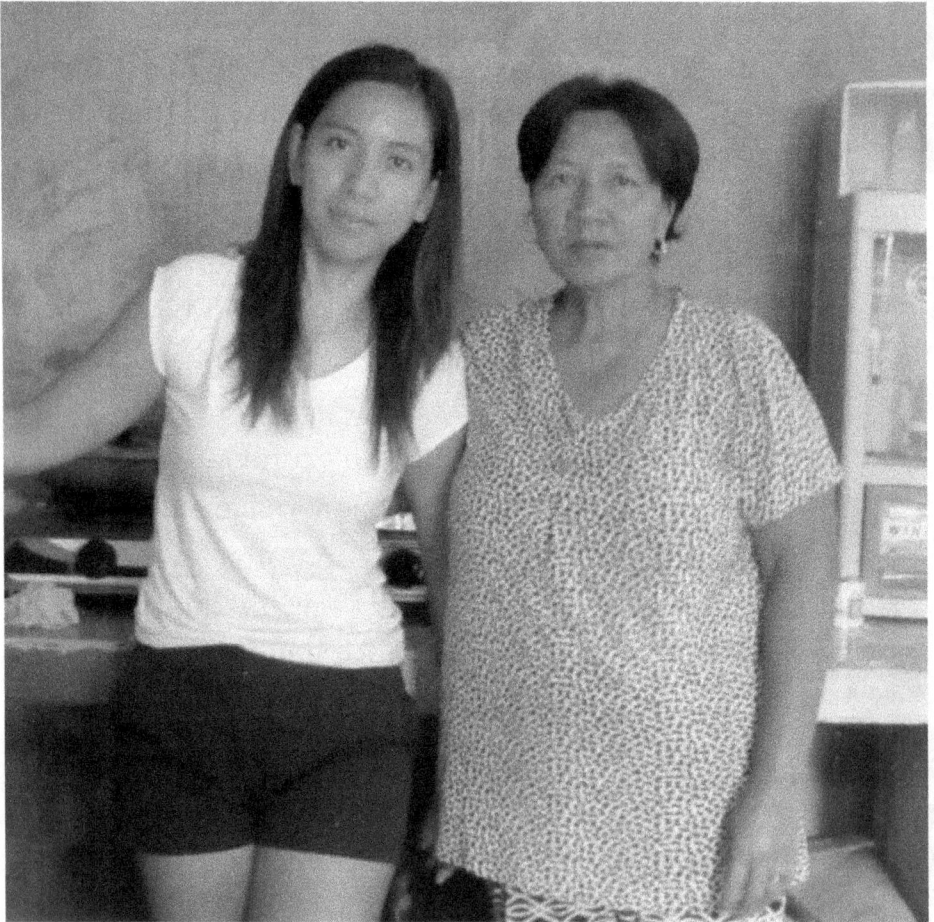

Chapter 3:
A Dreaded Diagnosis

Since then, I didn't focus much on my illness. One year later, while I was walking along, I spat up blood, thick and red. At first, I ignored it; I thought my gums were bleeding. After a few minutes, I spat again, followed by a loud cough. I was nervous, and I quickly asked my mom to check on the blood. My mom was worried, too.

The next day, I went to our community center, where they offered free check-ups. That day, I found out I suffered from tuberculosis — the dreaded TB. I had to face another challenge. I got this sickness due to charcoal's intense smoke. My father made it in a deep hole in front of our house. He would sell that to earn a living.

I told my dad many times not to make charcoal close to our house since every family member would inhale all the smoke. During the night, we couldn't sleep due to the thick smoke. But he didn't listen. After 15 years of making charcoal, my dad died from lung cancer and complications.

I want you to understand that even though my mom suffered from cancer, I didn't get my sickness from her. I realized that I got cancer because I was living in a terrible condition. I remembered my dad using strong chemicals and pesticides to spray our vegetables, fruits, and rice plants. He would pour the vegetables with pesticides at night, and the next morning we had to harvest them and soak them in the water for at least 30 minutes before we could cook them. Do you think those pesticides washed away? I certainly don't.

Sometimes we fall sick because of our environment and the foods that we are eating every day. So maybe I got my sickness from the food and the chemicals. We lived on a hillside, and I thought that the foods we ate were fresh. I didn't realize that we were also taking in potent pesticides and chemicals sprayed on them. I was still pretty young at that time. I understand now how vital these things are.

At a very young age, I had already experienced many illnesses, suffering, and pain. After cancer and tuberculosis, I managed to overcome everything. It's amazing! And I'm happy to say that my mom is still alive and healthy. I am grateful.

I was diagnosed with sinusitis while I was working in Saudi Arabia. It turns out I am allergic to dust. I suffered terrible headaches for about three years. I couldn't breathe well due to cysts that grew inside my nose. The moment I returned home, I went to the hospital to book an appointment to operate on me without spending much money. I remember it was precisely 4:00 am when I was queuing at the hospital to get a spot. So many people were there waiting! If I'm not mistaken, I was number 119. When I met the doctor, he said big cysts were growing close to my nostrils. After three days, I finally underwent surgery.

That's why my story is so important. It inspired me and countless others. It was a big lesson for me, and I am still here today. I am a very positive person; strong, energetic, fit, and healthy. That's why I embrace fitness. I am here today to share with the whole world that whatever happens in our lives, there is always HOPE.

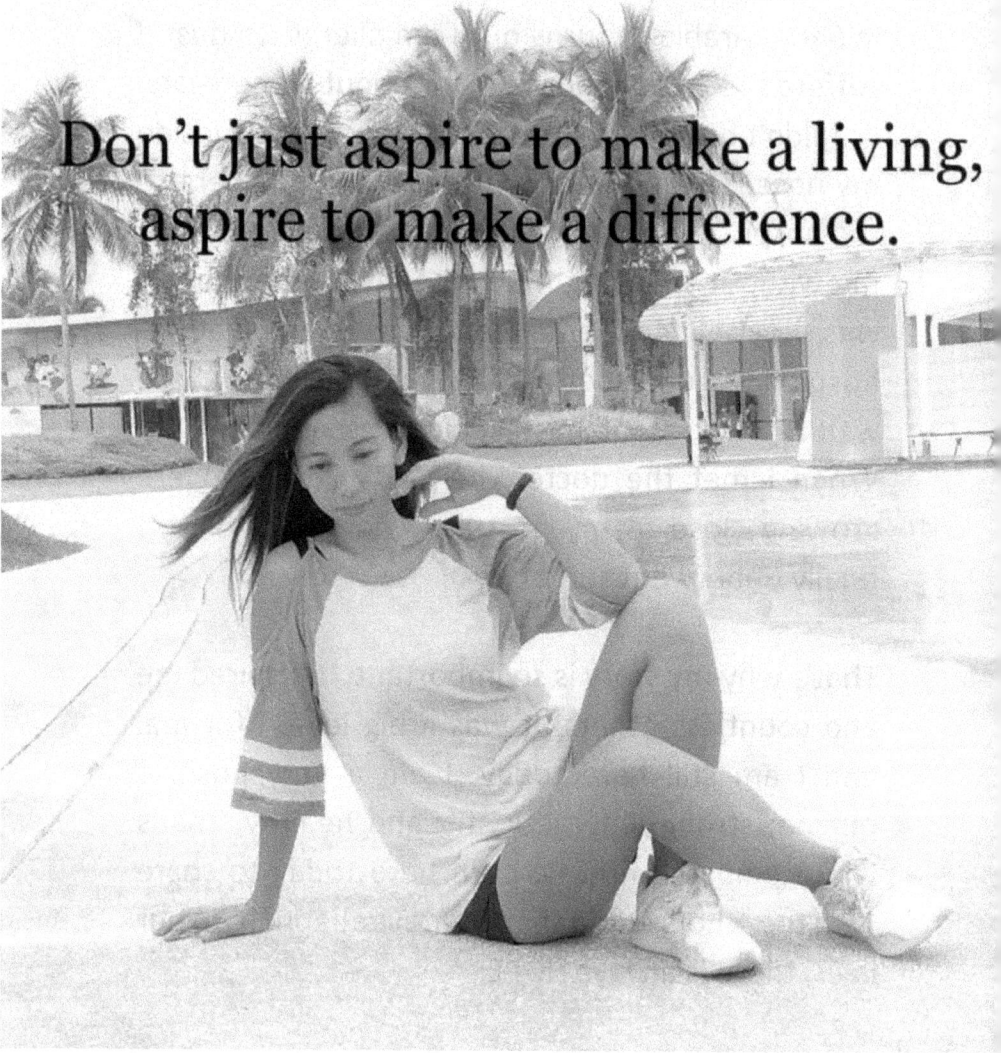

Don't just aspire to make a living, aspire to make a difference.

Chapter 4: Embracing Fitness and Good Nutrition

Since I have now embraced fitness and a healthy lifestyle, I feel like it is my responsibility to teach others how to take care of themselves, too. People need to understand what is in the foods that we are consuming every single day. My entire purpose for writing this book is so you can know how I overcame sickness and when and where I started embracing fitness.

I am proud and happy with my body's transformation, which has come about by working out. To those of you who are struggling with your weight and size or struggling to overcome sickness, I know for sure there is always a solution to these problems.

I have embraced fitness since 2010. I would do my workouts, but my nutrition wasn't that good. That's why I didn't see results until I hired a mentor, and he taught me exactly what to do. Since August 2018, I have taken this fitness journey very seriously.

I have been amazed by the transformation of my body.

I don't have access to a gym at all, so all of my work has been on my own. My goal was to tone up my body and be healthy, and I'm happy to say that I have succeeded. That's why I'm so excited to share this amazing transformation with others, especially with other mothers.

I am a mother of two beautiful children. I know the challenges. Let me help you get fit, toned, healthy, happy, confident, and strong. You will be amazed to be living in your new comfort zone!

I have gone from a size extra-large to a size small. I achieved this through my Mentor's help and guidance. I have learned that if you are not getting the result you want, something is wrong. You need someone to help you achieve your goal.

YOU CAN DO IT

Life is About balance

Chapter 5:

Learn from Your Past

My life has been like a roller-coaster ride, but before I start sharing my journey with you, I would like to share facts about me. I am a mother of two angels, like daughters. I graduated with a Bachelor of Elementary Education and grew up in the Philippines on Luzon's beautiful island.

I am writing this because I BELIEVE. I believe that sharing my journey will impact many lives, empower, inspire, and motivate others - especially if you are a mother who has been working very hard to support your family. If you have gone through a lot of hardship, pain, failures, and struggles in life, please read through to the end. I'm going to share with you how I overcame those pains, trials, and difficulties. I will teach you how to dream, develop ambitions, and create goals. Through this book, I will urge you to keep dreaming, keep working towards that dream, and remember, *IT IS NOT OVER UNTIL YOU WIN!*

I grew up on a mountain with my parents and siblings. I have fond memories of the days when I was young, even though the house we lived in was very poorly constructed of old wood with no stable foundation. On rainy days, rainwater will seep through the roof and flood our home. There was no electricity, and it was very far away from school. Everything was a long, endless walk – a walk to our neighbors, the market, and the city. We all talk about human's basic needs - food, clothing, and shelter, but my house was barely a shelter, and we were barely living.

No matter how poor we were, my parents still managed to feed us two and sometimes three times a day. All thanks to their inhuman hard work. I have witnessed with my own eyes just how much my parents sacrificed their whole life to feed their six children.

When I was eight years old and started understanding things, I realized how tough our life was. I helped my parents harvest corn, plant trees, plant sweet potatoes, cassava, bananas, and other fruits. If we need to survive, then we must help each other put food on the table. At this age, two of my siblings were adopted by another family because my parents were not able to send them to school. It was heart-wrenching. It still brings tears to my eyes.

Chapter 6:
My Elementary Life

I remember crossing a small river without the bridge to just go to school each day. My elementary school was unique to me and so much fun. I had to walk miles after miles to reach my school, but it didn't matter because I loved it so much. It was like a blessing that there was always someone there to help me across the deep-water river. But heading back home was a big hustle for me as I had to walk for an hour to reach our house on the hilltop. Despite all this, my mind was pure and innocent, so I enjoyed my walk in the rain back home. My life was so simple. I remember those days when I went to school without a lunch allowance. Sometimes I would drink water during lunch to dilute my hunger, and sometimes we were able to eat free fruit from our school backyard.

I feel my mother is such a blessing. She took care of us as much as she could. She sacrificed so much. I began to understand life at the tender age of 8. My father loved to plant vegetables and fruits. I have seen my parents wake up at 3 am to harvest, clean, and prepare vegetables. Mom sold all kinds of vegetables at a market. I helped carry the heavy things to the place where there was a Jeep that drove her the rest of the way. We were so happy to see her at the end of the day. Once my mom sold all the vegetables, she was able to buy nice bread and meat.

Since we didn't have electricity, we were all in bed by 6:30 pm.

My dad had farmland, but it was very far from our house. On the weekends, we walked about 4 hours to reach his land. He planted ginger, pineapples, bananas, corn, and different vegetables. I can't tell you all the hardships we went through with my family. The problem was a constant in our lives. Things were challenging, but it is inspiring to look back on those times now.

On another note, while in primary school, I received an award from our school. My parents were very proud of me when they heard the news that I was one of the top five honorable mentions in our class.

Chapter 7:
My Secondary Life

The secondary school was so far away that I could not travel every day to the school. At that point, I had to make a heart-wrenching decision to move out of my house and live near the school. That was the only way I could complete the school.

I remember the kindhearted teacher who was like an angel offered free lodging for the school children. Even today, thinking about that brings tears to my eyes. Kindness is rare, and if you find it, keep it and cherish it. I wouldn't be here if I wouldn't have completed my school, and the only reason I could afford to finish my school was because of the free lodging. In return for this kindness, I committed to helping my teacher with the household chores. Soon I became homesick as I missed my parents badly. I could only see them once a month due to the long-distance, and every time I saw them, I would break down into tears.

My mom was not keeping well as she went through so many illnesses in her lifetime. One day I got the news that my mom was hospitalized due to a heart problem, which shook me. She was my pillar, and I admired and adored her. She suffered due to insomnia, fatigue, and stress.

It has been a few years, and I have just started recovering from my mom's situation, and then I get another bad news that my dad's left foot began to shrink. It went to the extent that nothing could have been done, and finally, it had to be amputated to save his health and life. He wasn't a perfect father; he smoked, drank much alcohol, and a heavy coffee drinker. This combination took a negative toll on his body, which he couldn't come out of. Despite the challenges, he was still a hard-working father.

I secured a decent place to live, but I was still out of money, and my parents couldn't afford food money. I practiced going with very little food for days. Sometimes I'd have porridge, and other times just rice with water and salt. There were times when I ate nothing at all because I couldn't even afford the above. I completed my secondary school with only two uniforms. I take pride in saying that I was one of the top two in our class from the first year of high school to the fourth year. I did not let the circumstances shackle me. I push myself beyond the limit and got through.

Life can be extremely challenging at times, and it is like life is putting you to the test to see if you truly deserve happiness, wealth, and riches. People who are not passionate about doing certain things in life can barely survive this test as they end up giving up very quickly. I still remember that when I was young, I always felt that this is not how my life is going to end. I felt the Universe inside me, guiding towards an experience that only a few people dare to dream.

I experienced many challenges and hardships during those years. I faced many challenges every step of the way, but I committed to myself that.

"I will study hard and give my parents a better life."

Due to poverty, I would sell fruits and vegetables after school hours to make some money to buy ingredients for my food. It was hard enough, but I survived. I graduated from Secondary school with flying colors and dreams on my mind, but I couldn't afford to attend the university due to my parent's poor financial situation. My plan had to take a detour. But it was never tarnished. I was more determined deeply to figure out ways to develop myself and grow in my life. However, as I said, the experience can be challenging, especially to those who are doing things without any passion or purpose in mind.

I looked at many things, but unfortunately, nothing came to fruition. I couldn't find anything and the time was running out. The more I would delay finding a source of income, the more challenging every day gets. Someone suggested to me that I can make some money if I work as a helper. I had no choice, so without any further delay, I took on the job of a helper.

I remember working as a helper for a strict and fussy wealthy family with a big house. One day their teenage daughter threw her jeans on my face despite not having done anything. I was naïve and too scared to speak up for myself. I thought to myself that when I become successful and wealthy, I will never misbehave with others, especially those underprivileged.

The Universe has challenged me in many ways. While I was working as a helper, I fell sick. When I couldn't get better, I had to go to the doctor, and the news hit me like a speeding train. I was diagnosed with cancer in my neck. That moment I felt all my ambition and dreams fading away into nothingness. I can't remember what type of cancer it was, but I remember that a giant cyst grew on the left side of my neck and filled with pus. My body wasn't ready for any physical labor anymore, so I resigned from my helper's job and went back home to live the unknown days of my remaining life.

The doctor who initially diagnosed my cancer couldn't tell me exactly what type of cancer it was, so he referred me to a hospital in the City of Manila to get the second biopsy done. It took me a total of 8 hours to travel to the hospital from my home. We didn't have money to spend on anything like this; we barely had the money for food. Our money was all spent on basic survival needs with zero savings.

My Mom and I went back home with this news that engulfed us like a black hole, but my mom understood my situation and started chatting and laughing at silly things to keep me distracted and away from worrying. But I could see that she couldn't hold it any longer and was also getting sucked into this black hole of sadness and worry. My mother said, *"My daughter, we are so poor and don't have anything; where can we find this kind of money in such a short time? If we don't take action immediately, the cancer cells will spread to the rest of your body."* I could see the fear in my mother's eye.

When we got home, I burst into tears. I couldn't stop crying as I sat in a dark corner, thinking about how my life was about to end. Soon I was also diagnosed with tuberculosis, which crushed my mom and shattered my dreams. I couldn't believe that my life would end this way. I hated this situation, but one thing I hated more was giving up. After a discussion with my mom, she agreed to join me to visit our local municipality office. Looking at my situation and the medical diagnosis, they decided to pay for my tuberculosis medication. This was such a huge relief. Even though my problem was not over, this appeared to me like the light at the tunnel's end.

I traveled to Manila alone with limited financial resources. It was so little that my mother couldn't afford to join. I was a 16-year-old girl arriving in Manila to get another biopsy done. It was a long and lonely journey.

When I reached Manila, I was so nervous. I had no idea where to go, but I was brave enough to take this challenge. I asked every person I saw for directions. At last, I found the clinic. My first day in Manila's city was shocking it was so crowded; the streets were confusing; there were tall buildings; and so many cars and buses. I started to imagine things born out of fear. I was still innocent. Imagine yourself living on a hillside all of your years and never having explored life in the city. I felt so awkward and stupid for the first time.

I was so nervous about facing the doctor as he had this big needle, which he said he needs to put into the lump. I was scared of the bow and the needle. That was not a good combination. The doctor asked me to stay calm as he inserted the needle into the lump on my neck and filled the syringe with pus. The doctor asked me to call for the biopsy results after 48 hours. Since I had to wait in the city for another two days, every hour seemed like an eternity.

Chapter 8:
Searching for My Brother

During my stay in the city, I searched for my brother's address, where he was working with different families. His name is Jim. He worked as a helper in a beautiful house with six family members. I reached the address and met Jim after many years. I almost cried, felt wrong about my brother. He worked so hard. He washed all of their clothes, cooked everyone's meal, dusted the house, and did many more chores. I have no clue how he survived such an intense work life. He suffered like me. He used to wake up early to wash clothes and clean the whole house every day.

Years passed by, we experienced many ups and downs in our daily life. I remember soldiers staying in our house, which was expected to remain in private homes when patrolling in the area. Everybody in my house was afraid to say anything to them as we feared being shot. They had guns. We fed them our latest and limited stock of food even when we didn't have anything left for ourselves. We couldn't sleep as we were afraid of the soldiers in our house. When they were done, they left our little home. A few days later, around

3'O clock in the morning, we heard gunshots. We woke up, and in a panic, we hid underneath our bed for the whole night. The next morning, we listened to the news that my parent's friend had an argument with the soldier and was shot in the head.

Chapter 9:
My Parents

My dad was a very hard worker. He never took a day off. Every day he was up really early to sow the seeds of the crop. I remember him not sleeping at all at times when the moon was bright. He would take advantage of the glowing moon and plan to earn a living. My dad's favorite quote,

"Plant seeds now and you will have something to harvest soon. When you don't sow a seed, there is nothing to harvest."

After a long time, I got a chance to sit with my mom and talk as she was always working to put food on our plates. I remember her saying, "Who among you can make our life better? When can we have a better house? When can we move to a safe place and have many neighbors?" I kept quiet, but deep inside, I cried. I love my mom so much and wanted to help her have a better home. I committed to myself that I will make her dream come true.

Whenever my mom visited her siblings, she would bring back left-over food and worn-out clothes. We were so low that we couldn't afford new clothes, so we were thankful for the things we got which people wanted to throw away. If I wanted to buy something new, I had to pick up snails from our rice field for my mom to sell to the wet market (a place where perishable goods were sold). It was kind of fun to pick up small snails. One gallon of snails sold for 100.00 pesos.

I pitied my parents when I heard this next story. It occurred before I was born. My parents owned land, a farm about 1 hectare in size. This equals about two football fields in the US or about two and a half acres for the Western world. According to my parents, when my mom was diagnosed with cancer, they didn't choose other than to loan this land to one of our relatives.

They agreed that they could take back the farm anytime as long as they could come up with cash to pay back the loan. My dad's cousin decided. No written agreement was ever exchanged for the loan as they trusted each other. My parents were still the ones who took good care of the farm, but whatever corn or rice was harvested and sold, half of the money went to my parents, and the other half went to my dad's cousin. This continued for over 20 years.

My mom underwent chemotherapy for more than three months. She was admitted to the hospital, and they spent so much money. They also asked for help from neighbors and municipalities. According to my Mom, she almost died due to her brain tumor; the day of her operation was a miracle. She told me, "Prayers are mighty." After three months of staying in the hospital, my mom went back to our house. She had a long walk of more than 30 minutes to reach our home on top of the hill. After a few months, she was pregnant, and I was born.

Every member of our family worked really hard. We owned a carabao (a domestic water buffalo), and I was the one who collected rice straw or grass to feed her. It was challenging work. I had so many wounds, cuts, and scars from the sharp blades of the grass.

One more thing I can't forget: during rainy days, I had to collect drinking water from another hill far from our house. I carried a big gallon jug from hill to hill. It was heavy and difficult to maintain. Most of the drinking water in and around our home turned brown on rainy days, so it wasn't safe to drink.

I just want to include a note about my dad's addictions to coffee and cigarettes and his regular use of alcohol. I admired my dad because he worked so hard; however, he also got violent and slapped my mom over little things, like when he didn't have a cigarette. Cigarettes and coffee gave him pleasure - the only pleasure he could find in that hard life. He smoked three packs of cigarettes a day. To me, this was so upsetting! When he drank, he would get impatient and violent and throw things like plates, casseroles, and glasses at my mom's face or head. I got mad with my dad. One time, my mom ran away from us for three days. She couldn't stand my dad's attitude and behavior. Both of my parents were depressed and stressed due to family matters, financial hardship, and poor living conditions. As their children, we were severely affected, too.

Chapter 10:
My Siblings

The names of my family members are changed to protect the innocent ones. *

I recalled how strict my brother Bud was. I probably should not include him in this story, but he played an important part in my life. I remember how cruel he was towards me and our brother, Jim. After he graduated from Primary School, he seldom came to visit us. He was surrounded by imperfect people kind of like a gangster.

He was mean to all of us. If he asked me to wash his clothes, he counted to 10. If I weren't done on time, he would hit or kick me. I experienced terrible trauma and panic attacks every time Bud visited us. Even when I was sick, he punched my swollen leg. He would shoot me with a slingshot on my forehead. My forehead became red, swollen, and bruised. The worst thing he did was cut my hair to hide my forehead and the evidence of his meanness.

He told me not to tell anyone or else he would hit me again. I didn't say to my parents; they were away that day. Only Bud, Bill, and Donna were at home at that time. Bud was very bossy. In short, everyone was afraid of him. I didn't realize that he was on drugs at that point in his life. I even cursed him and prayed that he would die so our suffering would end. Even my mom was afraid of him.

One day, I was cooking lunch, and he suddenly picked me up and threw me down on the ground. He said he wanted to kill me. I was hurt and dizzy because my head hit the ground hard. I stood up quickly when I heard he planned to stab me with a long knife. My mother was screaming. She yelled at him, "Kill me - not Amanda!" I quickly ran to my sleeping father to get help, but I couldn't wake him. I chose to hide in the tall grass instead.

Later that night, I went back home. Mom was shaken but unharmed. Bud had already left and gone back to the place where he stayed. Years passed by, and Bud's behavior got worse. I told myself I would never forgive him.

One more thing I will not forget about Bud Bats use to be eaten in the Philippines when I was young, and we had to catch them. When Jim and I didn't see any bats during the middle of the dark night, Bud would kick us, punch us, and punish us. All through the night, Jim and I would be covered with mosquito bites. The next day, Bud took a long knife and said he planned to kill Jim. Jim quickly ran. The moment Bud was about to stab Jim, our carabao saved his life. A carabao is a domestic water buffalo kind of like a large family pet that also helped on the farm. Having massive horns also made her a formidable defender. Thank goodness the carabao was there in our backyard and was instinctively protective of us kids. The carabao was poorly injured by Bud and bled quite a lot, but she survived.

Chapter 11:
Off to College

I had a hunger for knowledge and was willing to do whatever it takes to get into the university, but my financial situation was terrible. My mom heard from someone that the priest in our church is willing to assist the youth who are willing to advance their education. I was filled with excitement and fear at the same time as I wasn't sure if I would be receiving it. A few days later, after applying to our church, I was called for an interview by the priest's secretary, where they asked me many questions about my intention, my desire, and my goals. Even though I vaguely remember all the discussion, but one answer is still engraved in my mind. When I become successful, I told them I would help millions of others like me, so they don't have to struggle. A few days after the interview, I was informed that the priest decided to support me. My mom's request was approved by the priest. Against all odds, when my dream was coming true, I couldn't believe it. Absolute excitement and happiness flooded my mind for the very first time.

No matter what, I was grateful to God for blessing me with this beautiful opportunity.

I always wanted to be a teacher, so the course Bachelor of Elementary Education looked very lucrative. I wanted to learn more about education and how to teach others. Even though I didn't understand the courses before my admission, I knew deep inside that this is the right option. Our priest sponsored my university fees. I also received a small allowance in exchange for cleaning the priest's secretary's office every Saturday.

My first year at the university was exciting but challenging. I stayed with my mom's brother, Uncle Agapito. It wasn't easy because I couldn't focus on my studies. I had to cook, clean, wash their clothes, and everything in exchange for paying rent to my uncle. I had to wake up early, around 4:00 am, to do the household chores. I often received a morning lecture from the neighbors because of the noise I made more first in the morning.

When I came back from university, I quickly changed my uniform and got busy with household tasks. I could only do my homework after 11:00 pm. It's not easy to be a working student. There was very little time for studying. Every Saturday, I had to visit the church and clean before they would pay the allowance. My life has never been easy, even when I was a kid. I have always worked as a helper in other people's houses.

Once every three months, I visited my parents. I saw my parents working very hard. Their routines were still the same: planting sweet potatoes, cassava, tomatoes, string beans, and other kinds of vegetables. We were lucky to have a farm. At least we had food to eat every day.

Chapter 12:
The Birth of a Dream

While I watched my parents work under the hot sun, I spoke to myself. I started to dream that one day, our hardships would end. I couldn't stand watching them work from 5:00 am to 6:30 pm under the scorching sun every single day. It was a painful feeling. Then suddenly, I questioned myself, why were there so many poor people? Those poor people become poorer and poorer while rich people become more affluent. What's their secret?

I went back to my Uncle Agapito's house. As usual, I had to work before going to my classes at the university. During lunchtime, I spent my free time in the library. I read books until my afternoon class started. One day, while I was on my way to my classroom, I saw my ex-boyfriend.

My Love Life – An Introduction

I haven't shared with you about my love life. We met in secondary school. After two years, I broke up with him. I couldn't have a relationship and

41

focus on my studies. A year and a half later, we accidentally met at the university. He was just passing by. He was happy and surprised. We smiled at each other. A few weeks later, I received a letter from him. I responded. We had no phones yet at that time. So we exchanged long letters. One thing led to another, and we became a couple.

Before classes started, I sold sweets to my classmates, so I earned the nickname "Sweet Seller." I was the funniest student in our study. I liked selling a lot. The problem I encountered was that I could sell, but I didn't focus enough on profits. I just enjoyed being a salesperson. I didn't need to spend extra money on my snacks and lunch. I got these selling skills from my mom. She liked selling our fruits and vegetables in the market ever since she married my dad.

When I was younger, my mom brought me to the market, and I helped her. I was happy to see all the buyers smiling. Our fruits and vegetables are sold so fast usually within 30 minutes. My mom always rewarded me for helping like ice cream or porridge. My mom told me to study well. She told me that I was blessed that my aunt and uncle were helping me now, but she didn't want me to forever experience that kind of life. There was no need for me to sacrifice so much and hard to work.

No matter how difficult my situation was during college, I survived. College life wasn't a comfortable journey for me. Sometimes I didn't have an allowance, and I missed some field trips and other activities. There were days when I sold products like Avon or Natasha to make some much-needed money. I sold bras, lipstick, shoes, and beauty products. I became a distributor. For the first year, the business was profitable. I received a commission and profits. I had many customers, too. I enjoyed attending seminars and events.

Then one day, I went bankrupt. Instead of earning money, I ended up paying for items taken by my customers. It took me about a month to spend the money I owed. I had no idea how to manage a business. What I knew was that I earned a commission for every item that I sold. Sometimes, I had to chase those customers to their houses to pay for the things they bought.

I can't forget the customer who owed me for sandals and underwear. When I went to her house, she was wearing sandals. She said she couldn't pay me because her son was sick all the time. I couldn't force her to pay me, so she gave me back the sandals that were already worn. What a headache! I'm glad I didn't ask her about the underwear.

I thought I could earn money selling. After one month of not paying my loan for the products, I received a summons letter. I was worried. I didn't know where I could come up with 14,000 dollars. My boyfriend was the one who received the message. He couldn't help me either - we were both students at that time. I promised to pay the owner of Natasha within three months.

After three months, I still couldn't come up with the cash. The lady came to the university. She threatened to file another complaint if I didn't pay her. My life was miserable - I heard painful words. I felt depressed. Every day, she came to find me, harassed me, and asked for payment. How could I pay her if I wasn't able to pay for my tuition? My answer to her was always the same: "I will pay you, just give me another chance. The customers never pay me."

I learned a big lesson from these situations. One day, my boyfriend asked me to stay with him in his apartment. I was in a mess, and I wanted to focus on my studies. I was in my second year of college when my boyfriend offered me some help.

A year later, I decided to approach my Uncle Agapito and asked him to help me move and be independent. I never mentioned my boyfriend to him. He agreed, so I promised that every weekend I would visit and help with household chores.

I was in my third year at university when I moved to my boyfriend's apartment. My parents had no idea that I moved out of my Uncle Agapito's house. When I visited my parents, I wrote a letter to my boyfriend. I forgot to hide this letter, and my mom read it. She was surprised and started screaming at me and crying at the same time. I asked her why she was crying. The reason why? She had such high expectations for me. She thought that I was the only daughter who could help them. I felt so guilty. I saw how disappointed my mom was. I lied, and I told her that I was working for someone else and staying with them.

One day I was surprised when I saw Linda (a friend of our family) on our campus. I tried to hide from her, but she had already asked some of my classmates what time I would finish my last lesson that day. When I was about to go back home, Linda spoke to me. I couldn't refuse to tell her the truth. She was furious at me. Without my knowledge, Linda had already gone to my boyfriend's university, where he was enrolled, and spoke to him about our situation.

That day my Mom and Linda already caught us being together in one apartment. My mom wasn't happy, and she collapsed. My mom suffered from cardiovascular disease. She didn't speak to me for a month. I was sad and worried, but I went back to my boyfriend's apartment. My mom never visited me. It took her three months to get over being angry with me. I asked for forgiveness, and at long last, my mom spoke to me again. She smiled. Finally, we chatted happily also, and I promised her that I would finish my degree. We went back to our apartment together with my boyfriend, my mom, and me. She wanted to see our apartment, and then she knew she could visit us anytime.

Chapter 13:
Becoming a Teacher

In my fourth year, I was finally thrilled. I had many friends, and I was surrounded by great and talented students. I was busy making my lesson plans and fulfilling the other requirements to graduate. There were many sleepless nights because doing lesson plans wasn't easy. I had to come up with great topics and lessons to deliver in front of the teachers. This year, I also started Practice teaching. It was exciting, though! It took six months to accomplish.

Every day, I had to get up very early as I needed to reach the school where I was assigned to teach. I was assigned to teach the 5th and 6th grades. It was fun teaching. All the students were disciplined and cooperative. They respected me, too. Some students gave me letters to show how grateful they were.

Days and months passed, but I was oddly distracted. I didn't realize at first that I was in the early stages of pregnancy. I was worried about how can I continue my studies? How can I face my students and my friends? My teachers and friends didn't even know that I was in a relationship. I told myself, I can't hide this situation forever. I decided to speak to one of our professors – a kind and gentleman. He advised me to talk to my boyfriend and settle our relationship as soon as possible. We decided to get married in a simple ceremony. My parents and my boyfriend's parents agreed to celebrate our marriage in the municipality.

I was wearing a maternity dress, going to Primary school to execute my practice teaching. Life was getting harder. Months passed by, and my tummy was becoming visible. My mom was so supportive; she visited me in our apartment, brought me a basket filled with fruits and vegetables. I felt so guilty that my mom needed to sacrifice because of my hard headedness. I promised myself that I would be able to help our family have a better life. This would not be an easy promise to fulfill because I was already in a young marriage.

It was finally time for our graduation. It was a fascinating time! All my sacrifices were to be rewarded. The same was true for my husband. He studied Criminology. I was assigned to teach Filipino subjects and Mathematics. I worked hard on my lesson plans. I used old typewriters since there were no laptops at that time yet. I would study until 2:00 am, and then I would get up at 4:30 am to make sure I delivered the lesson with excellence.

And then it came! The final day of practice teaching!

I was ready to face the teachers and my co-students, who would rate my teaching. I dressed up with a smile on my face and applied a little makeup. I was the second student who performed the learning. One of the strictest professors rated me in this practicum. I stood in front of students, teachers, and co-students. After the presentation, I sat and listened to the professor's feedback. I received great feedback.

The professor said:

- She has a clear voice that every student can hear easily.
- She produced excellent content.
- She delivered the material within the exact time limit.

- Students were able to cooperate with the discussion.
- She speaks with confidence.

Grade: 1.25. Yes!

[For those in the United States, this is an excellent grade similar to getting a 3.75 on a 4.0 scale.)

April 12, 2005, was our graduation day!

Woohoo!!!

Chapter 14:
Graduation Day

This is it! Finally, all my sacrifices will be rewarded. My brother, Jim, who was now a beautician in Manila, came home. He was so excited for me. He was the one who put makeup on my face and styled my hair nicely. My parents were so proud. All my brothers finished only Secondary school. I was the only one among all my siblings to earn a bachelor's degree.

Even though I was pregnant, I managed to study and graduate. I continue to be grateful to our priest, who helped me tremendously in my college journey. Without his help, I would not have been able to pursue any University education.

Our graduation day was filled with happiness. I saw how happy my parents were. My mom dressed up. She accompanied me on my graduation day. Two of my brothers were also there, but my dad stayed at home. He is not fun when attending events. He just likes to sip his coffee and smoke.

My mom said, "Finally, Amanda, it's your graduation day. If you hadn't entered into a relationship, you would now be taking your exams and applying for a job. Now you are pregnant, so you can only stay at home." I felt so guilty listening to my mom's sermon.

Chapter 15:
Life-changing Incidents

After graduation, since my husband didn't own a house yet, we packed our stuff and went back to my parent's home on the hillside. Two months after graduation from the university, I gave birth to a healthy and adorable baby girl. Having my first child was remarkable. She gave us happiness and also brought joy to my parents. My husband is a good guitarist, and he can sing well.

As usual, life was challenging. I am thankful for my parent's help because they were there to support my daughter and me. Neither my husband nor I had a job. We couldn't live without my parent's support. I had just given birth, and I was the one washing clothes, cooking, and cleaning because all of my family members were too busy only earning a living. We couldn't just sit idly and watch the baby grow.

Months passed by; life was becoming more challenging. There were times we didn't have enough food, especially during rainy days.

My Second Child

After one year, I was pregnant with my second child. I sighed to myself: I am such a failure as a human being. I couldn't stand watching my parents working in the sun because of me. I applied for a job as a Nanny, and my husband allowed me to work even though I was pregnant.

My employer was a Professor at Private University. She felt bad about my situation, so even though I was two months pregnant, she hired me. She had one son who was two months old. I questioned myself about everything. What a life. It wasn't easy.

I had to wake up early, clean their two-story house, prepare their breakfast, and cook lunch and dinner. About seven students also rented some of their rooms. Some of the tenants questioned me. Where's your husband? Why are you working as a maid even though you are pregnant? Some also said that it wasn't right for the baby if you do that hard. I was so embarrassed. I just smiled and continued cleaning, but deep inside, I was hurt and jealous of their happy and successful life.

One day, I approached one of the more mature students to watch the now 8-month old baby boy while I prepared my employer's dinner. Cooking wasn't my job. My employer's niece, who is also a student, was supposed to wash dishes and cook.

She was very lazy and used to put everything on me. The student was happy to help. I left the baby in his stroller and went down to the kitchen. The students were watching a movie at the time. While I was cooking, I heard a loud noise. I thought that something heavy had dropped on the floor. I was horrified to see the baby had rolled down the stairs from the second story in his stroller when I wasn't looking. I screamed. I thought the baby must have been hurt. It was a miracle that the baby was smiling. He was holding tight to his stroller and had no injury. I was shaking all over at the time. I didn't know what to do. Thankfully, the baby must have thought it was fun.

I was scared to tell my employer what had happened with the baby. When she returned home, she was smiling, so I took the opportunity to say to her about what happened. Then she quickly checked to see if her son was hurt. She said she would bring her son to the doctor for a scan.

Finally, everything was clear. I told my employer that I wouldn't let this happen again. I asked her to let me focus only on watching her son. No cooking unless she was there to protect him. She agreed and never got upset with me.

I often cried during the night time. I missed my daughter. Can you imagine? I was pregnant, and I was working as a nanny. I had a husband who had never taken any responsibility for his own family. It wasn't an easy job for me as I went through some sleepless nights. I felt like giving up, but if I didn't have a job, how would we survive? I questioned myself, why did I need to suffer like this? I was two months pregnant when I started working with this family of three. I visited my family twice a month. Whenever I was at home, my daughter was so happy to see me.

When I was with my family, I felt guilty about everything. I told myself: our suffering will end one day. After I give birth, I will make sure to get a better job. I was still blessed that I found a good employer who took good care of me while caring for their son. My husband was busy doing his own thing.

Chapter 16:
Christmas Celebration

My employer invited my family to celebrate Christmas in their home. They also asked them to stay the night. I told my family about my employer's invitation. They agreed, and they were excited about it. It was on December 24. My husband, daughter, and youngest sister came along. They stayed two days to celebrate Christmas with me.

My husband saw me working very hard. I woke up at 5:00 am to wash loads of dishes and clothes. He might have felt guilty watching me, but he didn't take any action. I didn't blame him for not having a job.

There were days when I was embarrassed to talk to people because of my situation. I was depressed, unhealthy, skinny, and I didn't look good at all. Some people thought I was 41 years old, but I was only 26!

After Christmas, my husband, daughter, and sister went back home. I was in tears seeing them leave, but I couldn't do anything. I had to work to provide for the needs of my family. One day, I had to go with my employer's husband to take her son for his vaccination. While we were on the bus, people thought I was his wife. I don't know; maybe he was embarrassed to hear those words. He was a nice guy anyway and younger than me. I didn't care about how they judged me. I was focused on doing my job. If I concentrate on negative thoughts, then I would end up staying on the hill and working in worse conditions under the hot sun.

Months passed by, and I began to have difficulties bending because of my pregnancy. I couldn't sit anymore to do the washing. I had to carry water from outside and bring it to the kitchen.

Some rich students approached me to wash their clothes, and they offered to give me some money. These students were still young, and they just loved to watch television sitting around after school. Another family approached me to ask if it was okay for me to accept their laundry. I agreed to all of it. So now, besides my monthly salary as a Nanny, I had extra money from doing laundry.

One of these families was my employer's relatives, so they were okay with it as long as it didn't affect my health. I was tired the whole day, but I didn't let anyone notice. When my employer asked me how I was, I told her I was okay. I was in bed every night by 10:00 pm and woke up at 5:00 am. On Saturdays, I always went back home to visit my family. I would use my salary to buy excellent food for our dinner, things for my daughter, and thank you gifts for my parents. Since they were the ones taking care of my daughter, they deserved to have rewards.

My parents asked me when I would be back since I was then in my 8th month of pregnancy. I didn't want to stay at home and get stuck in that environment. I told my mom, "I'll work another few weeks."

I got scolded by my mom. "You suffer too much ... the same as me. If you didn't get pregnant easily, then you could apply for a better job or work overseas. Soon you will have two children, and your husband doesn't have a job. He finished his bachelor's degree, but he doesn't even take the initiative to look for a job. You better take good care of yourself. Look at your appearance! You look old now and stressed. Once you give birth, make sure you use contraceptives and don't get pregnant again. I am the one sacrificing taking care of your kid."

I knew she sacrificed a lot because of me. I just kept quiet. I felt guilty and hated myself. In my mind, I promised to take care of my own family; though it's not a comfortable journey, I have to endure all the hardship. My parents were taking good care of my daughter, and thankfully she was a good baby. She was adorable, cute, and chubby.

When my dad came home from long hours of working under the sun, he quickly picked up my daughter and carried her around. I saw how happy my dad was whenever he held my daughter. The smile on his face, the way he made her chuckle. It was fun watching them laughing together.

When it was time to go back to my employer's home, my sister and my daughter walked with me to the place where there was a jeepney (a local taxi). While waiting for the jeep, I played with my daughter and chatted with my sister. My sister was only 13 years old. When the jeep arrived, I was in tears, leaving my daughter with my young sister.

Before I left them, I bought some unhealthy snacks for them. Back then, we didn't care much about which foods we ate. I didn't feel good about my situation, but it was the best I could do.

The moment I reached my employer's house, I quickly cleaned, cooked, and played with their son. I really appreciated them and was very grateful to have them during my pregnancy period. They were an awesome family.

The one who recommended me for this job was my aunt, the one I mentioned earlier because I stayed with her and my uncle while I was attending the university. Their house was only 10 minutes away from my employer. Whenever my Uncle Agapito or my aunt passed by, they smiled at me and waved. I smiled back, but deep inside, I was embarrassed.

Chapter 17:
Gossip – Painful Words

I heard some gossip. People said, "That's what she got after finishing her degree at the University." and "Amanda looks unhealthy like she's 50 years old." When I heard the gossip, I smiled, put my head up, and walked away. I tried to ignore all those words. Sometimes, I cried; it's okay to call to release all the destructive emotions inside, especially when people say painful words.

I had two more weeks left to stay; then, it was time to pack my things and say goodbye to the lovely family who took such good care of me during the pregnancy period. Working with them for those seven months made a big difference in my life. I learned a valuable lesson: focus on the child and not on cooking or anything else. I am lucky that their son didn't get hurt, or I would have been in deep trouble.

I learned how to communicate with different people, and last but not least, I learned how to be patient. The lady employer asked me to recommend someone who could be trusted and was hard-working like me. I recommended one of our relatives, and she agreed.

Kind Words from My Employer

My employer asked me to come back after I delivered the baby. She told me, "We like you so much. You are a very hard-working mom, kind and trustworthy. Please visit us whenever you want. You are always welcome!"

Wow! Hearing all these words made me smile and so very happy.

The next day, I went to buy groceries. I went out early since my employer's parents came for a visit to take care of their grandson. When I came back from the grocery store, I was surprised to see one of the students carrying my daughter. I asked, "Who brought her?" The student said, "Your Mom approached me to take care of your daughter since you were not here. She went to sell vegetables."

Oh, my God! I felt so bad seeing my daughter with dirty clothes and a dirty face as I was so embarrassed that my poor baby is suffering so much. It seemed like my daughter had never even taken a bath yet. I was sobbing then and sobbing now just thinking about it. My heart ached to see my daughter looking like that.

What's more, my daughter was sick with a runny nose and fever. I quickly cleaned her face and wiped her whole body with a warm towel. I couldn't stop sobbing while I am cleaning her. I whispered to my daughter, "I'm sorry. You shouldn't suffer like this. I'm taking care of someone's child, and it is meticulous. Even though you are my daughter, I can't take care of you."

Then my mom came. She handed me some vegetables to give to my employer. I saw how tired she was. Instead of scolding her for my daughter being so dirty, I quickly offered her a glass of water.

Poor Mom, she sacrificed too much because of me. Many nights she couldn't sleep, especially if my daughter wasn't feeling well. I thanked her for taking good care of my daughter and promised to make it up to her one day. They left after lunch. Of course, seeing them go made me cry. Life is full of challenges. We had been in poverty ever since I was a child.

I started to dream again. I whispered, ***"One day, I will help my parents have a better life."***

After delivering my second child, I decided to ensure that I never became pregnant again.

Last Day in My Employer's House

I had already packed all my things, cleaned the whole house, and prepared their meals before leaving them. Both of my employers came back from their jobs to say goodbye to me. Debra was already there (the one I recommended to work with them). It was time to say goodbye to everyone, and we hugged each other. Then the lady boss handed me an envelope with cash. I was very grateful for that kindness.

Finally, I could go home to my family. I didn't look back once I stepped out of my employer's door. I walked straight towards the jeep station and reached home at 6:30 pm. It was already dark. I wanted to surprise my family, including my husband. It was hard being back in a house with no electricity. I was used to opening the fridge and being surrounded by bright lights when working with a wealthy family. And now it was all dark. We were using gas lamps, and it was a very dim light. You wouldn't believe it. Our nostrils turned black from the fumes (which I really thought was funny). Many people experience life like this, especially when you live on a hillside so far from civilization.

Chapter 18:
Family - Together Again

It was beautiful to see my family's faces. We all looked haggard, even though we smiled. When one works so hard, especially under the sun, you always look 20 years older. That's the reality, and I had to accept the facts. This was only temporary. I knew that I wouldn't look like that forever. The next day, our journey began.

My husband and I moved to our own house that he built made of bamboo and wood. I opened a small store since our little community on the hillside was getting more populated. Though we lived in a small city with neighbors spaced relatively far from each other, we could still make money. We didn't make that much, but at least we could survive. Even no electricity, however.

I encountered the problem while selling fruits and vegetables because people owed me for my products, and they always wanted to pay a week later. Some neighbors were irritating because they promised to pay for what they took from my store, but they still had not paid me even after as long as three years.

They didn't realize that I had to buy the goods from a very far away market. I had to carry these heavy things and walk for more than 30 minutes. No car could get to where we lived. Finally, I closed my store. My capital was gone, and I went bankrupt. I chased people down and begged them to pay me back, but they did not. Other times, people were vulgar to me. They were the ones who owed me money.

In my home town, gossipers are everywhere. I learned to keep quiet. I wanted peace and not trouble. I suffered a lot while I was carrying my second baby.

There were many nights when my husband and I would fight, mostly when he was drunk. When I left my daughter while she was asleep, I couldn't stand his attitude anymore. He kept screaming, talking nonsense, and I couldn't swallow it any longer. He took the knife and kept saying he wanted to kill people.

I ran to ask for help from my parents. Our houses were only 10 minutes apart. It was raining and dark. Remember, we had no electricity yet. It was muddy, so I ran barefoot. I fell because there were big stones on the road. It was almost my due date. My mom was furious. She ran to check on my daughter, who was still sleeping. My mom carried my daughter back to her house through the rain and the mud. She scolded me so badly. She asked me, "How could you be so irresponsible and just leave your daughter alone?"

I told my Mom I didn't know what to do anymore. I was tired of working for the whole day. I didn't sleep well since my husband wanted me to wait on him, serve him, give him food, and set the table late. He wasn't all that bad. It was just when he was drunk; then I couldn't stand his attitude.

My daughter and I stayed at my parent's house. After an hour, my husband was screaming outside. He wanted me to come out immediately. My dad was furious and yelled back at my husband, "You better get away from here. We were sleeping, and you are screaming at 3:00 am! Such a disrespectful person you are! Go away, or else I won't forgive you."

Luckily, he listened and went away. I was upset and stressed, that's why the next day, my daughter and I stayed with my parents. My husband didn't bother us. We didn't talk or see each other for three days.

These events made me think. I should have listened to my mom. She said that marriage at an early age would probably give me a headache. She said that I shouldn't get married so young. Regret is always at the end of that road.

We really couldn't avoid arguing and felt like life was complicated. Not having money was also a big reason for not having a happy relationship. My appearance had become terrible as my skin was dehydrated, and my face was skinny and ugly. I remember one of my siblings telling me, "Hey, Amanda, you look about 55 years old now." I responded to him, "Hey, I look amazing then. I think I look over 65!" He laughed with me.

Whenever I looked at my face in the mirror, I was sad. I saw how skinny I was. I told myself, you won't be like this forever. You looked beautiful and fresh when you were a teenager. I couldn't even afford to buy beauty products for my face. Of course not!

I could hardly afford food - how could I afford to buy things for my skin?

Now my advice to you if you have read this far and you can relate to my story, you better think a hundred times before entering a marriage. Make sure that the person is the right partner for you. Every one of us wants to be happy. I still considered myself happy because, during those hard times, my parents and my children were with me. They were my saviors and my heroes. They helped me take good care of my children and myself. Without them, it would have been difficult to survive.

Chapter 19:
The Day I Delivered My Baby

It's always good to be prepared in life, especially when it comes to delivering your baby. My tummy started aching. It was almost my due date. My dad went to get the midwife since most mothers in our community gave birth in their homes. The midwife came about six hours before I delivered my baby. It was a pleasure to see my newborn baby with the cutest little face.

No matter how I struggled with pregnancy, I was blessed with two beautiful daughters, even though I worked hard. They have the most beautiful faces and perfect skin. After birth, we stayed with my parents. I know that my parents loved me then and still do now. They took such good care of my daughters and me.

My husband was also busy trying to earn a living, but no matter how hard he worked, it was never enough. If I convert his earnings to Singapore money, he only made about $6 per day. In US Dollars, that would be about $4 per day. Without my parents' support, it would have been hard to survive. My parents provided my children's milk.

One week after giving birth, I started to clean the house, wash the clothes, and do the cooking. In our tradition, you should rest at least one month before going back to work, but because everyone was busy, I didn't choose to do the household chores. A few weeks after giving birth, I became sick due to a lack of rest. My mom stayed at home and took care of us. While I was walking in our backyard just to take a break, suddenly I felt dizzy and collapsed. I knocked my head on the ground. What was the reason why I collapsed? Lack of rest and sleep! You were lucky if you were married to a responsible husband. I'm not blaming my husband at all. This was a choice that I made. Being born into a low environment can affect one's decisions in every area.

As I mentioned during my secondary and college journey, I was forced to be independent at a very early age. I didn't even see a doctor when I collapsed; I couldn't afford it. Life just kept getting harder and harder. It affected me physically, mentally, and emotionally.

One day, my husband received a call from a friend and was offered a Manila City job. He was excited, and he quickly processed all his documents. A month later, he traveled to Manila and promised to give us a better life. I stayed with my parents, together with our two children. After two months, I start receiving money from my husband. It wasn't all that much since he needed to pay for his lodging, transportation, and food, but at least it was something.

My daughters were getting sick quickly due to charcoal's smoke right in front of our house. We were all affected because of the smoke. My dad dug a hole in front of our home, threw in all the broken fresh wood, and covered it with soil. It took much hard work. My dad cut the wood in the forest and carried it to our home. He moved heavy branches even though his left foot was amputated, and he had a very skinny body.

To be honest, I couldn't stand seeing my dad in this state. I wished I had a job to support them so they could experience a happy life. I would sit in a corner and imagine good things. I prayed that one day someone would offer me a job. But I was insecure. I didn't look good; I looked skinny and old.

Tiya Dely

I am fond of listening to the radio. There was a program that I liked called "Tiya Dely." For Filipino people, Tiya means Aunt. This auntie was already 70+ years old, and she was able to talk clearly with an energetic voice. She sounded about 30 years old. I wanted to see her in person. I admired her a lot.

In her program, she shared tips on how to be healthy and live a longer life. She gave suggestions on what to eat to be fit. She also gave advice. People would send her letters asking about their love life, family matters, and other things. Every week, she chose one winner offering money for the best story. I can't remember the exact amount.

I Googled Tiya Dely to learn all about her. As I wrote this on October 2, 2018, I found out that she just passed away last month on September 1. She was a Philippine radio broadcasting icon well-loved by generations of listeners and advice-seekers who tuned into her radio counseling programs.

In her program, I learned how to cure cancer in a natural way mentioned earlier in this book. She advised one of her listeners to eat boiled potatoes and carrots every single day for six months. She urged the patient to consumed only two kinds of vegetables. Miraculously, it worked, and the patient became cancer-free. Isn't it amazing? You might be smiling at this moment while reading my story because I wrote to Tiya Dely. I sent her a long letter telling her all about my family's journey, about how we lived in a dark forest and everything, but I don't know what happened to my letter. I didn't hear back from her, or maybe it was lost. But trust me, I wrote the exact name and address given by Tiya Dely. It was that important to me.

Win a Prize of P1500

There is another radio program I listened to called DZRH. We didn't have a television well; we didn't even have electricity at that time. It says, "Win a prize of P1500!" They picked ten winners weekly for the raffles. Requirements: Send any Nestle wrapper, put at least ten pieces in every envelope, and send it to the radio station. I was excited to try anything.

Here are the things I did to collect Nestle wrappers: I went out to pick them up from the garbage located anywhere in our backyard, our neighbor's backyards, and in a muddy park-like area. It was fun collecting those wrappers. On our hillside, most of the neighbors threw their garbage anywhere. Rain or shine, I picked up and collected all the Nestle wrappers I could find. After collecting hundreds of them, I washed and dried them to look new and clean. After that, I sealed them in an envelope and sent it to the address given.

My mom laughed at me and said, "You're funny doing all these things. Thousands of people are joining in that promotion. Do you think it's that easy to win?"

I told her, "You never know! Maybe I'll be the lucky one out of 1000 senders (I was laughing). I am dreaming to have an income."

Sadly – I did not win.

The Charcoal Pit

I was bored with my life! No income. There was a time I wanted to buy shampoo or some beauty products, but I couldn't afford to. Due to our lives and our town's difficulties, people got sick quickly, including me, my mom, my kids, and my dad, because of the dirt and the smoke. Most of the people were making charcoal. Most people don't realize that making charcoal produces much smoke before it turns to charcoal. Every day, we inhaled the super thick smoke produced by the charcoal pit.

I told my dad that he shouldn't make charcoal in front of our house because it caused us to have bad health, especially my young children. Sooner or later, we will all suffer from lung cancer or breathing problems. My dad didn't listen. He had done this for years. We used wood to cook our meals. I mentioned before that I was diagnosed with tuberculosis. I never smoked in my entire life, but I suffered all these chronic diseases due to our low lifestyle.

The illnesses were caused by constant inhalation of smoke from an open wood fire used for cooking. The main complaints of "wood smoke-associated lung disease" are cough and dyspnea (difficult or labored breathing) with bronchial obstruction. Since people in our town rarely recognized the risks of wood smoke inhalation, they hardly reported their exposure.

One day while our family was busy harvesting charcoal, we saw someone walking toward us. We didn't recognize who it was since we were sitting under the bright hot sun. Our eyesight was a bit blurred - too much sunlight. It was my mom's sister, Aunt Tina. We were all happy and smiling to have her visit us. She brought a lot of food, like bread, meat, and snacks. She's my favorite Aunt ever. She helped us a lot.

Aunt Tina asked me, "Amanda, I came here to ask you if you want to work abroad? They need someone urgently." I was so happy and excited. Then my parents asked, "Amanda, do you know how to speak English?" I laughed and answered my dad, "Of course, I can speak it, but only simple English." Then Aunt Tina replied, "You don't have to know a lot of English because even those in the Middle East speak only simple English. You'll be fine as long as you know how to clean and cook."

We harvested charcoal after 5 hours of chatting about working abroad. Tina also helped us. All our fingers and faces were completely black. Next move, we need to find a buyer for our charcoal. It only cost P60.00 per sack at that time; if it's in the Singapore dollar, then about $2 something. Our life cycle had not changed for many years, making charcoal, planting vegetables and fruits.

We experienced the most challenging difficulties in life on Earth.

However, we never gave up.

Chapter 20:
My Life as a Helper

I'd been asking for guidance and help from our Almighty God, that he would send me a person and use this person as an instrument to make our lives easier. He heard my prayer. I told myself, "Thank you, Lord, for sending my Aunt today to convey such good news." This was my lifelong dream to have a monthly income so I can help my parents.

Now we had a new challenge: Where can we find the money to process my papers? It was going to cost us a lot of money to process a passport and transportation for traveling to Manila, and then, even more, to travel to the Middle East.

We had a carabao that helped my dad carry heavy stuff from faraway places. My parents sold our carabao just to have the cash to process all my documents. I felt bad about it. However, my dad said, "It's okay, Amanda ... we will buy her back once you receive a salary." They found a buyer for our carabao after about six days of searching.

I've been crying while I typed that last part. My dad passed away six years ago, but this is how I remember him. I made a commitment to myself. I will never give up earning a living until I get what I want, and I see my parents satisfied and happy with their lives. I will make my parents' well-being the priority in everything I do.

This is the funniest thing you might read in this part of my story: my parents had the mistaken idea that once someone worked overseas, that person became famous and rich in our community. This still makes me laugh today. The reason why I mentioned this is because my parents had seen many foreign domestic helpers or people who were working abroad have the resources to build their houses, buy cars, receive big boxes of goods and fancy stuff. They started to dream about these things for me.

After one month of processing my documents, the Saudi Arabian family from the Middle East called me. I was nervous because I thought I wasn't able to communicate very well - I mean, in terms of the English language. This was my first time speaking to someone from overseas. I was still naïve and inexperienced even though I had earned a Bachelor's Degree.

While processing my documents, I encountered lots of ups and downs since I wasn't aware of much in Manila City. Mary, a friend from our town who had been working in Saudi Arabia for a long time, recommended me to work with her employer's newly married daughter and husband. Her sister Lina accompanied me to the agency where I could submit all my requirements. She wasn't that close to us, so I didn't feel comfortable talking to her. We traveled to Manila, with all of our expenses paid for by me, including our hotel, transportation, and food. Lina wants everything perfect, and I had to take care of everything since I owed them for this journey. As soon as we reached Manila City, we went to the agency where I could submit all my documents. The staff there wasn't friendly at all. I wondered if the reason they didn't show me any respect was because of my looks. As I mentioned before, I look like an older woman with a skinny body and a skinny face with dry skin. I was 25 at that time but looked 42 years old! We stayed in Manila for at least five days. We were told we only had to stay for two days, but the agency mistakenly gave us the wrong details. It was upsetting because

I did not have enough money to stay longer and would have to spend more to buy the delicious meals that Lina demanded. It was my responsibility to feed her. She would ask me if I want to eat this or that, but I just told her I wasn't hungry and I didn't like the food. I didn't have enough money to spend, so I pretended to be okay. I bought only water.

Since we had three days more left to stay in the hotel and I didn't have enough cash, I called my mom via telephone and asked her to send me money. They were worried about where to get cash again. They made a way to send me cash. They went to a loan person lending money with 10% interest. The next day my mom sent me money via LBC. I withdrew the money together with Lina. That day Lina said she needed to go back home because she brought only three days of her medication. I gave her cash for transportation and cash for her meals while on her way back home. I was left alone in the hotel. I went out to see the surroundings. It wasn't a safe place because it was too crowded. People were busy selling on the streets; drunkard people were everywhere. Snatchers were everywhere. It was a scary place for a young woman walking by herself.

While I was out walking in Manila, a man approached me. He spoke in English, and I thought he was an American guy. He told me his name was Mark and that he was visiting from the United States. He asked me to help him. He said that he was robbed in a taxi and they stole his money, passport, and phone. They even stole his necklace. I thought to myself, this is weird!

The Scammers

I remember what my mom said, be careful around the people you meet in Manila. There are people who are scammers. Keep all your things safe. Keep your money inside your shoes. He kept following me as I walked to a mall, telling me a story about his life in the USA. He begged me for money in order to go to the police station to file a complaint. He followed me for three hours, asking for money. I got irritated and stayed away from him. He kept following me again and again until I gave him P50.00 (the equivalent to SGD 1 dollar 50 cents). He wasn't satisfied with that and begged me for some more, and I told him I didn't have anymore. I told him I had to skip lunch because of him. He thanked me and ran away. I followed and observed him. He was running so fast. That's when I realized I got cheated – he was just another scammer. I went back to my hotel. I sat down, and I told myself I was stupid. I was so embarrassed to reveal my stupidity that I never shared this story with anyone. Especially my parents, because I knew they would scold me. I learned a lot of lessons regarding this event. I got cheated, and I never ate lunch, but at least I wasn't hurt. For that, I was able to smile at the end of the day.

Hard Decisions

Applying for a job overseas is very challenging. My daughters were still very young. My first child was only two years old, and the youngest one was only eight months old. My heart hurts every time I looked at their beautiful faces. I left them with my parents while processing all my documents. I am very thankful to my parents that they were still alive when I decided to earn a living overseas. I wanted to help my parents a long time ago before I decided to work abroad as a helper. I had already promised them to help them to experience a good life one day. It was my 4th day of staying in Manila alone. My husband was working so he couldn't come and see me yet. I couldn't stay in his apartment because he had roommates. I went out again to relax. I went to the mall where I could see lots of different things like bags, shoes, clothes, good food, et cetera. I told myself that one day would be able to afford to buy good things for myself and my family. There were families having fun together, having lunch together, playing together. I started to imagine being like them one day. I wished my family was rich, so we didn't need to suffer.

I kept walking until I reached the 7th floor. There, I met a few applicants who were applying in different countries like Hong Kong, Singapore, Cyprus, Taiwan, Malaysia, Dubai, New Zealand, and many more. We chitchatted for about an hour. Some discouraged me not to apply to Saudi Arabia because there were lots of abuse cases that hadn't been solved by their government. Others said most of the employers there were very strict. Others told me that you couldn't talk to any men there, and you have to cover all parts of your body, including your face. You have no days off. Another applicant said her friend was already working in Saudi Arabia for about one year. She was doing fine, and her employer treated her well. I told them that I was recommended to my new employer through a family friend. As a directly hired applicant, I shouldn't have to worry much. We had lunch together; we shared lots of our burdens and experiences in life. We were the same, and all came from poor families. After lunch, we went out together from the mall and walked together towards the agency building, since their agency was also the same as mine. I went up to the agency unit. There I sat and waited for my turn. I waited at least three hours; there were many other applicants. Some staff was very nice, and some were really rude.

Finally, it was my turn to be interviewed by the Saudi Arabian owner of the agency. I was nervous; my palms were cold and sweaty. He asked me many questions that were written on my biodata (resumé). After the interview, he looked me into my eyes and said, "Don't worry, Amanda, you will have the best and kindest employer in Saudi Arabia. They are a young couple. Okay, now you can go back to your hometown, and my staff will keep you updated. Prepare all your things. In about two weeks, we will book your ticket. See you, Amanda, and have a safe trip." Hearing what he had said comforted me, and I was happy. I packed all my things to go back to my hometown. I chose the cheapest bus since I was alone. While waiting for the bus going to my home, I observed many people selling different kinds of foods and stuffs like boiled eggs, chips, newspapers, toys, water, and other things. In Manila City, it looks like if you work hard, you can surely survive. There were so many ways to earn money since the population is crowded and growing. I just kept quiet in a corner, looking around. There were people picking up cans of Coca-Cola, bottles of Sprite, and more drinking bottles or soda cans. These people woke up so early just to pick up those cans to sell. I asked one of the ladies how much she earned per day. She said P15-20.00. That's equivalent to SGD50 cents (or 35 cents in the US). It depended on how many cans she could collect the whole day. Mostly she dug in very dirty muddy trash. Like me, she had to endure so she could survive.

I fell asleep. After 2 hours of waiting for the bus, I was awakened by those working people I had been watching. I was afraid there would be no available seat for me with so many passengers, so I rushed up and managed to be one of the first in the queue! It took us seven hours to reach our destination. I slept inside the bus. I was traveling at night time, so I could get home around eight in the morning. At every petrol station, the bus driver stopped for a stopover in order for us to get food or drink. I would stay sitting down and rolling my eyes at the people around me. They seemed to have money. I was hungry, of course, but I didn't have extra money to buy anything. "Poor Amanda," I whispered to myself.

At last! One more station, then I can get out of this miserable bus. If you sit too long on a bus, you don't feel energetic at all. All my body parts were aching. I quickly went straight to a tricycle for the next leg of my trip. For those who do not know, a tricycle in the Philippines is a motorcycle with a sidecar used for public transportation. I was on the tricycle for 30 minutes and still had another 30 minutes of walking time to get to our home. My total traveling time from the hotel to home was ten hours and twenty minutes. I was exhausted and tired. Finally, I reached home, and I saw my kids and my mom. I washed and changed.

My mom was so happy, asking how everything was in Manila. I happily responded to her, "Mom, in two weeks, I will be flying!" I could really feel how happy and excited my mom was. We were chitchatting nonstop and dreaming about the future. She reminded me a million times to be honest and good at all times with my employers. There were more rules, like: Never answer back. If you see some wallet or money or maybe a necklace, do not touch it. Your employer might be testing you; inform them quickly.

Then my mom also told me, "I was also supposed to work abroad when I was 19, but your dad wouldn't allow it. We could have had a good life then."

I reminded her that if she were working abroad, then I wouldn't be here. We laughed together. No matter how simple and hard our life was, we needed to smile, laugh, and feel the essence of life. My biggest inspirations are my kids, my parents, and my whole family. I'll work hard in order to pursue my goals.

I was grateful to be flying very soon. While waiting for my flight, I kept myself busy cleaning our wooden house. While cleaning, I found out that our house isn't strong enough to last too much longer as one of the pillars of our house already sunk due to too much water that pooled during rainy days. I began making a list of the things I would settle once I started receiving a salary. I have another two sisters to help. They were both in primary grades. Still, there was lots of money needed to spend. I had to help my mom with her regular check-ups due to cardiovascular disease—sigh o many things to settle. I had to face all these since my two eldest brothers already got married and had their family problems. And my dad's addiction is horrible.

He was smoking heavily and addicted to coffee. There were times that I was worried about my children. My mom wasn't stable enough to watch my kids, and she collapsed many times in the day. I told my mom, "Ma, please prioritize your health once we have money. Go for a proper check-up and ask for proper medication. Once I start earning, change your glasses so you can see clearly. Please bear with my kids as I promise you, I'll bring abundance to our family."

I had one more week left to spend with my family. My parents were both busy on our farm, planting vegetables, making charcoal, and the usual tasks. That week was also the time to harvest rice. The rice is harvested by cutting the rice stalks using a sharp sickle. My Dad and my Mom went to our farm together with three people. I stayed at home and prepared and cooked snacks and lunch for everybody, including meals for the workers. My kids both behaved, thankfully, and I finished cooking on time. At exactly 11:30, the workers and my parents came home with sweaty faces and dark skin. They were so hungry and tired.

I reminded them that we were going to ask one of our neighbors about seven minutes away from our house to use their mobile phones. We couldn't afford to buy a cell phone yet at that time. Our neighbors had relatives from overseas. That's why they could use mobile phones and had electricity. When a call came for me, our neighbor would come over with the message. My daughter's dad called informing us he was sending money and everyone was happy.

The problem I encountered with the neighbor who lent us the cell phone was that she overcharged us with SMS and receiving incoming calls. We were ignorant at that time with no idea about how to use a phone, especially for sending messages. It's true I was new to this technology, so this neighbor charged us P50.00 every text - equivalent to $SGD1.50 or $1.05 US dollars. Too much, right? But of course, we couldn't complain because we were asking them.

It's great to examine the behaviors of people around to make me motivated and inspired. No matter bad or good, I still considered it a good inspiration. No matter how tough our life was, we knew how to respect and value people. I am grateful to our neighbor because, without her, we couldn't communicate by phone. Our neighbor received a text from the Saudi Arabian Agency. She quickly came to our house. She was more excited than us! She was still far away from our house, but she was already screaming with excitement and out of breath when she reached our home. "Amanda Amanda Amanda, you have to get ready and travel to Manila as soon as possible!"

I had already packed all my stuff one week ago, so I didn't need to hurry up, finding all my things. I began to feel sad thinking about not seeing my family for two years. Even though I've been away from my family since I was in Secondary school, this time was different. I felt nervous, excited, sad, and happy. I definitely had mixed emotions. I comforted myself by knowing this was the answer to my prayer a long time ago. I was ready for this journey. I knew I could get along well with Saudi people. I thanked our neighbor for her kindness and the effort that she spent during the processing of all my documents. She always ran to my house to bring me my messages when I got them, even during those times that she was busy washing or cooking. I owed her for this. I included her also in my list. She will have something from me one day. This is our belief; once a person does something good for you, you have to do something great for them in the future or pay it forward.

I had another two days left to be with my daughters and family. That night I couldn't sleep. I kept sobbing and hugging my daughters.

Even now, while I'm typing this story, I had to grab tissues just to wipe away the tears. As of today, I am still working as a domestic helper, and while I'm writing this story, I am currently working in Singapore. But don't worry, I'll tell you about my situation here in Singapore. I promise you; you will be amazed once you find out about my story. I am sure every reader will be inspired and motivated, and you will be applying some of my tips to take action in your everyday life.

The next day, it was time for me to say goodbye to my daughters, parents, and two sisters. I felt extreme pain from the bottom of my heart. My dad was holding my youngest daughter while smoking and drinking coffee. My daughter had the 'flu and a runny nose and was jumping in my dad's skinny lap.

My daughter was only eight months old, and the other one was two years old. I couldn't stop crying. I hugged my mom, my daughters, and the rest of the family. I walked away, carrying my luggage, without turning my head. I can still hear my eldest daughter crying while I was stepping towards the zigzag road with lots of rough stones and mud. The road to our home wasn't made of cement or any kind of hard surface. During the sunny days, it was all dried dirt, and during rainy days, it was all mud and water. Rocks that fell from the hills were all over the place. It brought us nightmares, but I swear we lived and survived for the past 30 years.

As I am writing this, the tears are still flowing. Remembering the past makes me a better and stronger person anyway. I am not who I am without those experiences, without those challenges and struggles.

Chapter 21:
Time to Go

I left early since my mom's sister was dropping me at the bus station together with my Uncle around 10 in the evening so I can arrive in Manila in the day time. I spent almost my whole afternoon at their house so I could relax my mind. They are the kindest relatives ever. Since we were kids, I remember how kind they were to my family. My Aunt gave me a lot of advice: be good with my employers, cooperate with other helpers just in case I will be meeting some helpers in the future, be mindful of my words, be respectful to all the people whom I'll be meeting there, follow instructions given by employers, and don't complain. I responded, "Aunt, thanks for all the advice. I will remember everything, and I'll be the most obedient helper in Saudi Arabia, then we can both be laughing together." I had my dinner there. My Uncle cooked my favorite meal, meat with vegetables. My Aunt and Uncle said, "Amanda, don't be shy, eat all you can... see how skinny you are. You need the energy to travel tonight."

That night, I spoke to my husband, and we planned to meet at the bus station located in Manila City so we could say goodbye to each other. He was not able to drop me off at the airport since the Saudi Arabian agency staff would accompany me. My Aunt and Uncle brought me to the bus station. All the buses were totally full. We saw some buses with standing passengers—all packed. No tickets were available yet this time. I told my Aunt and my Uncle, "I can manage myself to get a bus." They refused to leave me alone. They wanted to be sure I was safe. We waited for more than two hours!

Around 1:00 a.m., there was a bus going exactly to my target location. It was challenging to get a seat. It was the last bus for that night and packed with many passengers. The driver said I would have to wait for the next bus around 4 a.m. My Aunt begged the driver to let me on and said that my flight was later that morning. The truth was, my flight was the next day. My Aunt was so caring and worried that I wouldn't reach Manila on time. The driver let me sit in front where there was no seat. I would have to sit in a small space for 7 hours. I didn't choose at that time, and we already waited for more than three hours. My Aunt said goodbye to me, and they both hugged me. I saw my Aunt in tears. She cared so much about my family. "Take care, Amanda, and don't forget to write us a letter," I responded to them. "Aunt, Uncle, please visit my parents if you have time. I'll repay you one day, and I will not forget your kindness." I went in inside the bus without turning my head. I didn't want to cry again inside the bus, and I didn't want people to stare at me.

There were so many people on the bus, and I prayed that someone would get off at the next station so I could relax my back and sleep. No passengers got off at the next station. We all had the same destination. Imagine 7 hours of travel in an uncomfortable sitting position. I had cramps in my feet, body aches, and a headache. It was tiring and frustrating. When I reached the final destination, I saw my husband with sleepy eyes. When I told him about my situation inside the bus, he was very sad. Before he dropped me at the agency, we had breakfast together, talked a while, and he shared with me about his job. His manager promoted him to a security officer, and his salary increased by 2%. I advised him to support our kids and give extra to my parents since they were the ones taking care of our kids.

After breakfast, he dropped me off at the agency, and we said goodbye to each other. I went up with my luggage, nervous, but with excitement. When I reached the agency, one of the staff said, "Hi Amanda, finally you are flying tonight. Congratulations and good luck with your new employer." The owner of the agency spoke to me and told me all the dos and don'ts. "Once you reach Saudi Arabia, you have to wear a uniform that your employer will give you. You have to wear the niqab (a garment of clothing that covers the head and face of a woman leaving only her eyes exposed), and don't talk to any man. Be good to your employer so they will treat you nice. Don't go out without your employer with you, don't use their house phone without their permission, don't watch television, and many other things." I promised to be good and to comply.

When it was time to leave for the airport, one of the agency's staff accompanied us. Since I don't have any devices with me, I asked the staff to call or text my family. I gave our neighbor's mobile number to let them know I am flying in a few hours. I was nervous, having no idea what Saudi Arabia looks like, but I was curious about how people treat other nationalities and want to explore more.

There were seven more confirmed applicants with us going to the airport. When we got there, the staff guided us to the queue and where to wait for our boarding passes. We waited there for at least two hours. I said goodbye to the staff member who accompanied us; she was kind, and she wished us luck and reminded us to take care of our belongings - especially our passports. My tears began to fall. I told myself, "Yes! I am flying, and this is it! I can start to fulfill my dreams, to help my parents, to give a better future for my children, and to save money for myself." Then I told myself not to cry anymore and walked into the airport, brave and strong.

I sat in the waiting area where passengers waited for their names to be called. When I heard my name, my heart began to pump fast (I'm laughing while I am typing this part) because it was my very first time flying in a plane. So exciting, isn't it? I entered to find my seat. I took only a few clothes with me since I can't wear shorts or blouses in Saudi Arabia. The plane started to fly, and I started sobbing again. The guy beside me seemed to be a traveler, good looking and wearing name brand clothes. He looked at me and asked me if it was my first time working overseas. He offered me some napkins and told me not to worry, that I would be all right there, and to always think positive. It was a relief to have someone motivate and inspire me. I did stop crying. It took us more than 10 hours of travel. I slept on the plane with an uncomfortable back and suffered from a headache. If I had a book to read then, it would have been fantastic, but I wasn't a reader at that time.

Chapter 22:
My Journey in Riyadh

Our first destination was Dubai Airport. It was a great experience for me, seeing many great and wonderful things and all the bright colors that filled the surroundings. Dubai International, recognized as the world's busiest airport for international passengers, offers more than enough in the way of distraction, entertainment, and indulgence to while away the hours between connecting flights. I walked and explored by myself while waiting. We stayed at the Dubai hotel for one night before heading to Riyadh. I met a few Filipina. My roommate was a 45-year-old lady who talked nonstop about her job in Qatar as a female tailor. While she was talking, I fell asleep. The next day, I went to the hotel's dining area in time for breakfast before leaving Dubai. It was clean, with so much nice and healthy food. It was all self-serve, so I choose the foods that I hadn't tasted before. I ate only a little while others kept going back for more food. It was my first time, so I was quite shy. When you come from a poor family and have never experienced eating in a restaurant, it is hard to act naturally. I can smile now and admit I was ignorant at the time.

Then it was time to get ready for the bus that would bring us back to the airport so we could continue our journey to Riyadh. The two other passengers were quiet and busy staring at the surroundings, while I was busy observing people around me. Dubai was foggy and cold, and I wondered if my body could get used to staying in such a cold place.

Riyadh – So Much Sand

I didn't know that Riyadh was one of the hottest countries in the world and gets many sandstorms. I discovered that during my stay, which I'll share later. I waited for 1 hour 30 minutes for the plane that flew from Dubai to Riyadh. The flight lasted one hour and 55 minutes. The moment the plane landed at the Saudi Airport, my heart began to beat fast. I was a mix of emotions - excited to see what my employers looked like and nervous to see them, but finally at my destination: Saudi Arabia. I took out my passport and scanned it. Then I collected my luggage.

I was surrounded by a mix of different nationalities like Sri Lankans, Indians, and Indonesians. It was crowded. We all went to the waiting area where we could wait for our employers to pick us up. Some people had cell phones and called to update their families. I approached one of the Philippine ladies and gave her our neighbor's number to let my family know that I arrived safely.

After 4 hours of waiting, my name was called to announce that my employer was there to pick me up. A lady from the airport accompanied me to meet the employer. There I saw him, neatly dressed wearing a thobe (or thawb), which is a long garment similar to a robe and considered 'Arabic dress.' He was young with muscular looks and greeted me with a welcoming voice, "Hi Amanda, how was your long trip? Did you sleep well? Did you eat well?" I told him, "I didn't sleep well, Sir, but I did eat well. This was my first time traveling overseas, so my body is still not used to it, but I am good."

He brought me to the car park where his wife was waiting. There I saw my lady employer wearing an abaya and a face veil, and I could only see her eyes. She introduced herself as Zara and offered me some water. I was thirsty and grateful for the water. She asked how to address me, and I told her she could call me Amanda. I always addressed her as "Ma'am." I told her I was happy to finally get to Saudi Arabia and meet them. We chatted in the car for the next thirty minutes. I always referred to her as "the lady employer" in my head. It was as if she didn't have a name in my mind.

We reached their big house, and the moment their garage opened, my eyes opened almost as wide. Oh my God – their house was like a mall! I felt a sudden sadness and just wanted to go back to the Philippines. I took my luggage out from the backseat and followed them inside. I looked at their very dusty garage and the large backyard. When the lady employer took off her abaya, I was very surprised to see that she was pregnant! Mary, who recommended me to work with them, didn't mention that she was pregnant. She mentioned that they were newlyweds. I was disappointed to not know this ahead of time; it would mean more work for me.

The lady's employer told me she was expecting to give birth that month. I said, "Oh! Mary didn't mention that you are expecting a baby, Ma'am."

She just smiled. She showed me around their house, and I got another surprise: I would be working and serving two families! I kept quiet, but deep inside, I was wondering why Mary didn't tell me any of this. Then the lady employer showed me my room, on the top level close to the rooftop. They seemed to be a nice couple. She was only 17 years old, and the husband is 19. The lady's employer handed me clothes to wear every day. She also gave me an abaya to wear whenever we visited her parents or went to the market. She also handed me a niqab - a garment of clothing that covers the face. She asked me to put it on as soon as I changed.

Don't Ever Talk to Men.

She gave me instructions on what to do and their policies. The first thing that I remember that day was when she told me not to ever talk to her husband. If I knew he was already awake, I was to stay in the kitchen and close the door. I was also told to cover my face every day. She told me she would be upset if I was not wearing the niqab, but she told me in a friendly way. She gave me instructions on how to clean and wash their car and clean the dusty backyard with water. I quickly got changed into the uniform she gave me, covering my face like I was supposed to. I felt uncomfortable, but I know I should respect their culture.

This was my first time ever washing a car. It took me 1 hour 30 minutes. Their backyard took me 3 hours to clean. It seemed that nobody cleaned it for a year; you could scoop the dust. It was thick!

That first day was challenging for me. I was thirsty and hungry. The lady's employer came out and asked if I was okay. I told her, "Yes, Ma'am, I'm fine here. It took me too long to finish because it's dusty, and I had to carry the pail with water just to wash the floor."

If you are a first-timer working in a different country, having to deal and communicate with unknown cultures, you will feel sad and tired so fast. You have to adjust to everything, but you can't complain. You have to be observant and obey everything they ask you to do. Be alert at all times. I was shivering while brushing the floor; it was cold outside. My lips become chapped and dry due to exposure to the wind and cold air. When I was finally done, my hands and shoulders were sore from using the broom for five hours.

I went inside and started cleaning their living room right away. I was tired and very hungry, but they didn't offer me any food yet, and I was too shy to ask. Since it was my first day, I felt I had to work like crazy, so the employer would be impressed. Around 9:00 p.m., the lady employer called me and offered me a home delivery meal of a double Big Mac with cheese and a large Sprite. I worked from 2:00 p.m. to 9:00 p.m. without rest or food. I sat down in the kitchen to eat, staring at all the kitchen appliances. I wondered if I would be able to operate all of those machines and how I was going to clean the high wall. Take note: If you don't have electricity or own any appliances in your home, you will need to adjust yourself or study things that are new to you. When I worked for different families in the Philippines, they didn't have such machines. I told myself not to worry that I would learn what I didn't know and would not hesitate to ask for help. How different things are today when you can Google anything you want to know!

After I finished my dinner, I quickly cleaned up the table and started working again. At 11:00 p.m., the lady's employer told me I could stop working and could continue tomorrow at 5:00 a.m. I was to clean the living room first and have her husband's breakfast ready at exactly 6:30 a.m. and make sure I closed the kitchen door. "Don't also forget to polish my husband's shoes. Once the garage is closed, then that's the only time you can be out from the kitchen." I told her I would follow her instructions. Before we ended our conversation that night, she taught me how to operate the washing machine. Their washing machine was very high tech and different from what I had ever seen or used in the Philippines.

Later that night, I showered with cold water since the heater wasn't working yet in my room. The water was cold. It made me shiver. My room was very wide and big but had no windows. The bed was small with a very thin mattress. There were small drawers where I could keep my clothes. I unpacked my luggage and then stared at my pictures of my daughters and my family. I couldn't stop sobbing; I missed them so much. That night all I could think of was seeing Mary – the one who recommended me to work with these families. I hadn't seen Mary in person since I was a kid. I set my alarm clock for 4:00 a.m. and went to bed.

I didn't sleep well that first night because I wasn't used to the climate. My employer said winter would end in two months.

I made sure to be up at 4:00 a.m. since I was scared that I wouldn't finish cleaning their wide living room with lots of expensive decorations and other stuff. When I heard my alarm, I quickly got up, washed my face, and brushed my teeth. This was the funniest part of being a beginner helper like me; I thought getting up early and making much noise cleaning here and there made your employer impressed. Their stairs were made out of steel; when you wiped the stair fence, it echoed throughout the house. I continued cleaning until 5:00 a.m. with the broom since I couldn't use the vacuum yet. The couple was still sleeping. With every swipe of the broom, there was more of the same loud echo. The lady came out of the bedroom and said, "Hi, Amanda, you woke up so early. We can't sleep with all the noise. I told you to get up at 5:00 a.m. Next time, don't clean the stairs first; just clean the living room and kitchen." I responded, "Oh, I am sorry, Ma'am. It won't happen again." She went back to sleep.

The Second Day in Saudi Arabia

When the lady employer got up, she made a list of what to prepare for their breakfast. She didn't know how to cook since they had a helper since she was young. She handed me a recipe book. They just moved out of their parent's house a few months ago. After we chatted and I prepared her breakfast, Cindy came in. The lady employer introduced me to Cindy, the one who stayed in the same house but with a different door. That day, I had more of an idea that there were two families to serve.

Bear in mind that most Saudi homes are much larger than western homes. Even apartments are much larger than typical apartments in the West. Additionally, the climate in Saudi Arabia requires daily dusting and sometimes several times daily, vacuuming and mopping, especially during the sandstorm season. I said to myself after our conversation. Oh, my God! I hope my body can take it. The house of my employer alone seemed too much for me to manage, but two houses with the same four stories! It was a lot to do, with their big guest rooms. And both had cars (I have to wash the cars too)! I already had a lot to do with having to learn their foods; they are a bit complicated.

The lady employer and Cindy seemed to be nice and sounded friendly when they spoke to me. I told myself that it was fine to work long hours as long as my employers treated me well. Once our conversation ended, I quickly started cleaning from 8:00 a.m. to 11:30. Then from 11:30 - 12:30, I had to cook lunch. For the first time, I touched their stove (I was a bit nervous). I cooked pasta using a recipe from her recipe book. After cooking, I served her and Cindy, who can come only if the husband is not around. In Saudi Arabia, a lady can't talk to any men, including a brother-in-law or cousins.

After lunch, I went to the other house to start cleaning. Stepping into that big house for the first time caused me a terrible headache from all the dust everywhere around the house. I didn't even know where to start. Cindy showed me where to find all the cleaning stuff. Her kitchen was very unorganized. There were dirty dishes everywhere, but that made me realize that she knew how to cook, at least. I started cleaning their living room first, then their Bedroom, the toilet, and then the kitchen. Since there wasn't time to clean the whole house that day, I cleaned only the important parts. Cindy thanked me. I was surprised at how sweaty I was that day, even though the weather was cold.

I went back to my employer's house and saw the lady employer sitting in their living room watching her favorite show. What a good life she had! I quickly went to the kitchen to have a glass of water. I continued cleaning. That day, I didn't finish working until midnight. My body was tired and numb. I wasn't expecting to sleep well; I had a long plane ride only the day before and was likely suffering from jet lag. How I wished my employers gave me a few days to adjust to the new environment and let me gradually become familiar with their houses and routines.

I went up to my room and sat down in my bed to relax my back before I took my shower. I was already thinking about giving up. My fingers were already very dry with cuts, and the detergent I was using was very harsh. I was thinking about Mary. I wanted to see her as I needed someone to talk to to express my mind. It was 1:00 a.m. I went outside my room and slowly opened the rooftop door to where I dried the clothes. I couldn't see anything with all the high walls around me. I went back to my room and tried lying down in bed, but my eyes were wide open. I took out paper and pen and started writing to my family, to tell them about my first day experiences. I fell asleep while writing.

I woke up again at 4:00 a.m. That second day, I only slept for two hours. My body still couldn't adjust to the weather. As usual, I prepared omelets, fresh orange juice, and toast for the male employer. This time, I already cleaned the stairs slowly with no sounds. When the lady employer got up, I asked her for gloves because my fingers began to crack and bleed. She had to ask her husband to buy them for me because he was the one who bought the groceries. Helpers aren't allowed to go out without employers.

Days passed by, and I slowly adapted to the weather, the work, the people's attitude around me. No matter how tired I was, I still managed to smile - especially when both of the employers showed appreciation for my work. They liked the way I managed everything, except for the cooking.

After three weeks, the lady's employer told me to get dressed in my abaya. She was going to bring me to her parents' house, and I would be able to see Mary. "Really, Ma'am? Thank you so much!" I exclaimed. At last, I would see Mary in person. The lady's employer was surprised; she thought I already met Mary in the Philippines.

I quickly changed into the abaya; it was uncomfortable, but I had to wear it. The driver came to pick us up. Her parent's house only 15 minutes away from their house. My heart began to beat fast. I was very excited.

When the gate to her parents' house opened, I saw Mary cleaning the playground. I ran down from the car with tears in my eyes and quickly hugged her. I couldn't stop crying. I was happy that I saw Mary, but my feelings were mixed. After helping her clean their wide playground, I began to understand why she didn't tell me I'd be working for two employers. In the Philippines, I couldn't have imagined having to clean a wide basketball court. I began to feel bad about her situation; their house is bigger than my employer's house. We talked non-stop while we cleaned together. Then we went to their kitchen, and she offered me some coffee and a biscuit. Since we were staying for dinner, I helped her cook. That day I learned a lot from Mary. She taught me about cooking and gave me tips on how to manage my time so I can take a nap during the day.

The lady employer introduced me to her mom and sisters. They were nice. Around 10:00 p.m., we went back home. I was more energetic and motivated than before. That night my employer didn't make me work anymore, so I went straight to my room and went to sleep early.

When I got up, I noticed I had a fever. I let my employer know that I had a fever and suffered from terrible headaches, runny nose, and high fever. She gave me Panadol to take, that's all. (Panadol is known in the US as acetaminophen and works as a pain reliever and fever reducer.) I learned that day that even if you are not feeling well, you have no choice and still need to perform your duty as a helper. I went to the other house to clean their garden and garage. I was tired and feeling lethargic.

Chapter 23:
A Baby Girl

After two months, the lady's employer delivered her first baby. It was a girl. Right from the moment she gave birth, my schedule became more hectic. I had more guests to serve, too. I slowly learned more about their culture. If one is married into a Saudi family, this can mean having many guests in their home. I learned the proper manner of serving tea. Almost every day, her Mother-in-law came and showered the baby.

I repaid my debt to the agency after two months, and finally, I had my first full month's pay! My employer happily asked me where to send the money and how much. She also offered to let me call my family. I gave our neighbor's number, as usual, who ran to my family. Before I called, the lady's employer told me I could only use the phone for five minutes because calling from Saudi to the Philippines costs a lot of money. I was waiting in front of her while she was dialing, and finally, my mom came to the phone. I missed them so much, especially my kids. My mom told me that both kids had been hospitalized recently, and that made me really sad. Then I told her, "Mom, I finally received my first month's pay! I'll send it to you all. Thank you for taking care of my kids."

I couldn't stop my tears when I heard my kids' voices calling "Mama ... Mama!" It was painful to be away from them. Before ending the call, I told my mom, "My employer treats me well, and my work here is okay. I can manage everything." I didn't mention any hardship, so she wouldn't worry. She was already sacrificing so much taking care of my kids. I wanted to talk longer, but my employer was staring at me to signal me to end the call.

Months passed by. I overcame boredom by working continuously. Four months after the baby was born, the lady's employer enrolled at the University. I then had to take care of their daughter by myself. I had a very busy schedule. They gave me a baby monitor with audio, so I was able to work while the baby slept.

The lady employer told me to be prepared for the hot summer coming soon. Sandstorms attack Saudi Arabia, and I would have to keep all windows and doors closed at all times. She told me not to hang any clothes outside and to wear a mask, especially when I'm outside cleaning and watering the plants. I thanked her for the warnings and advice.

The lady's employer always asked me to do her homework. She thought I was clever and smart. She read my resumé and knew of my Bachelor of Elementary Education degree. I often answered her homework questions, and there were times I went to sleep very late because I had to answer her essay homework while she was busy watching her favorite TV show.

Filipina Attitudes – Co-Helpers

Once a month, I had a chance to see Mary when they gathered for a family dinner in her employer's house. There I slowly figured out some of the Filipina's (a Filipino girl or woman) attitudes and behaviors towards each other. Every time my employer brought me to different houses, like in her parent's house or in-laws' house, I had to cooperate with the maids and not the employer. It became a game of Helpers versus Helpers. Good conversations could turn bitter. Helpers that held their positions for many years would boss around the helpers that hadn't been employed as long. If I had to stay the night in a place with such a helper, I could not go to bed without working like a donkey. Clean this, clean that it seemed non-stop. Even if I wanted to sit for a bit and drink some coffee or have snacks, the co-helper would follow me and tell me I couldn't. Some would even lie and say there were cameras watching us.

Once, we stayed for two nights in another house. I wasn't happy, because helpers who didn't work together didn't communicate well. I just kept quiet and did my things without talking to them rather than argue. So even if I was hungry during that time, I pretended to be all right and just drank lots of water. I wanted to boil an egg for my breakfast, but this tiger helper wouldn't allow me to cook. Terrible attitude!

While I was cleaning the guest room, I almost collapsed. I could feel my body weakening while I was removing a heavy curtain using the tall ladder. But I continued to work no matter how hungry and weak I was. I learned from that day, dealing with co-helpers can be challenging. I didn't mention these events to my employer because I wanted peace. I slept with little food in my stomach. Sometimes it's tough to pretend to be okay in front of co-helpers because we all share the same room.

I didn't understand that instead of building good relationships with each other, they chose to be bitter. We all are far from our families and loved ones. We are only able to see our country once in two years. I would think we as helpers would want to treat each other nicely while we are so far away from our families.

I get dismayed staying in a different house, but I have to endure everything. I didn't have the right to complain as Riyadh wasn't a safe country at all. I have to cooperate at all times with helpers and employers. Once we reached home, I would quickly drink lots of water and eat fruits, and be thankful I was home. I would rather stay alone than deal with rude people. I can do my things in peace.

Chapter 24:
Celebrating Ramadan

I had no idea how Muslims celebrated Ramadan, so when the lady employer asked me if Mary had explained Ramadan to me, I told her that she had not. The lady's employer then explained to me about fasting, what to cook, what time they have to eat, and what time they have to pray. And then she added, "So please pay attention to these as we don't want you to walk in front of us while we will be praying in the living room. One more thing, you have to go to sleep very late as we have our meals at midnight."

Ramadan is the ninth month of the Islamic calendar. It is a time when Muslims around the world focus on prayer, fasting, giving to charity, and religious devotion. The last third of Ramadan is a particularly holy period, as it commemorated when the Quran's first verses were revealed to the Prophet Muhammad. Muslims believe it was during this month that God revealed the first verses of the Quran, Islam's sacred text, to Mohammed, on a night known as "The Night of

Power." During the entire month of Ramadan, Muslims fast every day from dawn to sunset. It is meant to be a time of spiritual discipline — of deep contemplation of one's relationship with God, extra prayer, increased charity and generosity, and intense study of the Quran.

It's a time of celebration and joy, to be spent with loved ones. At the end of Ramadan, there's a big three-day celebration called Eid al-Fitr, or the Festival of the Breaking of the Fast. It's kind of like the Muslim version of Christmas, in the sense that it's a religious holiday where everyone comes together to exchange gifts and share big meals with family and friends. I wrote down everything my lady employer told me about Ramadan on a piece of paper to make sure I wouldn't miss anything. I was nervous, of course, knowing I needed to prepare many kinds of foods for two families and guests. And I have to respect their beliefs and culture.

Days and weeks and months passed, and suddenly there were changes in their attitude towards me. The lady employer was always suspicious about their daughter's safety. One day the lady went to attend her class and left her daughter under my care. During lunchtime, I had to cook lunch for the lady employer and Cindy. While the baby was still sleeping, I quickly went to the kitchen to cook their lunch. While I was cooking, I saw someone walking outside the kitchen. It was weird because that's not the way for entrance nor exit. The moment I saw the shadow of the lady's employer, I heard the door open from Cindy's room. I was completely shocked when Cindy flew into the kitchen, followed by the lady employer. They wanted to find out something that day, but I'm not sure what. At the same time, the little daughter woke up because of all the noise. The lady employer started screaming at me about leaving her daughter alone. She also started yelling insults. "No wonder you became fat in just a matter of months! You eat too much!"

Oh, my God! I hadn't eaten my breakfast or lunch since I wasn't able to cook. I told her I was just preparing the ingredients for their lunch while the baby was asleep. I explained that I had to prepare the ingredients ahead of time to make it easier for me to cook since it's my first-time celebrating Ramadan.

It's not easy having lots of work and then having to cook different kinds of foods you are not used to for one meal. That day, she didn't talk to me. It was a big mistake for me to leave their daughter alone in her room. Even though I apologized to her and nothing happened to their daughter, she still wouldn't talk to me. I kept quiet to let her cool down. I learned a lesson that day. For three days, she didn't talk to me even though I greeted her in a nice way. Remember, during Ramadan, Muslims shouldn't hate anyone. But the lady employer kept hatred in her heart towards me.

Chapter 25:
Sandstorms

I couldn't stand the dust from the sandstorm outside. The clouds get extremely orange, and super thick clouds of dust fly outside all over Saudi Arabia. No matter how many times you wiped the windows or vacuumed the floors, you couldn't get rid of it. Even if you used one finger to touch the thick curtain, you could see the dust flying in the air. Their backyard was even worse. I suffered every time I cleaned even though I wore a mask. My nose would bleed, and I would get terrible headaches almost every day from the dust.

I appreciated the other couple; sometimes, they helped me clean their playground and garage. The only thing that I didn't like was that whenever I cleaned their room, Cindy would be there watching everything I did. It was very irritating, but that's the way some employers are, and I have to respect it.

One day, I remember when the lady's employer gave me a blue uniform. It suited me well, and I looked good in that light blue color. When I first arrived in Saudi Arabia, I was tanned with a skinny body. After eight months, I had become chubby with a round face, and my tan lightened because I had to wear those clothes that cover my whole body from head to foot. After I put on the blue uniform, I was surprised when the lady employer suddenly asked me to change and give back the uniform to her. I asked her why, and she said she accidentally gave me the wrong uniform. But I wasn't that dumb; I noticed something weird in her facial expression when she saw me in it. That day, the male employer was there, and it was the second time I saw him since I arrived. He said, "Good morning, Amanda." I greeted him back since he came to the kitchen to take their daughter. The baby had been crawling around while I was washing dishes.

When the husband left, she quickly confronted me and scolded me for responding to her husband. This was the second day of Ramadan. She got upset with small things. I went upstairs and changed. I washed the blue uniform so I could hand it back clean. I said to myself, and I have to be patient and never answer her back.

Chapter 26:
I Became A Butcher

My schedule was busy. The male employer brought lamb meat that needed to be chopped. Lamb and goat top the lists of meats preferred for evening meals. It took me almost four hours to chop the lamb. Can you imagine chopping a whole lamb by yourself? At least two whole lambs without ahead. I didn't have experience as a butcher in the Philippines, especially for a whole lamb, so it took me a long time to finish. In other countries, you have to learn everything before you apply as a helper.

That day I was very tired from cooking, cleaning two houses, cleaning two kitchens, taking care of the baby, washing clothes, ironing, and doing whatever else needed to be done. The moment I went up to my room, I almost collapsed. It was hard going to bed after 2:00 a.m. knowing I had to get up at 5:00 a.m. I had no energy during the day, especially because I got right up and immediately started my chores. I admit sometimes I didn't have time for myself; there were days I didn't shower or brush my teeth! If you were in the same situation, I'm guessing you would do the same with only two to three hours of sleep and no rest during day time.

After a few weeks, we went to the house of the employer's parents. They have to celebrate Ramadan there. That day I saw Mary and the rest of the helpers. Their house is bigger than the church in the Philippines, with great big playgrounds (bigger than a basketball court in the Philippines). They had many guests, so all of the helpers were busy serving every guest, working non-stop. Mary told me Ramadan is the busiest month, but not to worry; I would get rewarded after Ramadan. That night I was just observing how they celebrate the holiday. These families belong to one of the richest in Saudi Arabia, so most of their things are expensive and luxurious. They prepared the most expensive foods. We went back home after 1:00 a.m. My body was weak and tired, and I wanted to rest, but I couldn't because I still needed to iron.

Chapter 27:
Helper's Day

One month full of doing the same thing over and over can be tiring for helpers in Muslim countries. We called the end of Ramadan "Helper's Day" because it was the day we would receive money from employers and other members of the family. Yes, it's true! On the last day of Ramadan, all the family got dressed nicely in new abayas and new niqab.

The next day, the end of Ramadan, it was time to show generosity to poor people. I was washing plates when the lady's employer handed me 100 notes, including Cindy. The lady employer was smiling and happy; I hugged her the moment she handed me the money. There were other guests who gave me money, and I collected a few hundred riyals.

A Saudi Arabian Riyal is equal to about .26 cents in the US. I was the happiest human being on earth. The moment I counted the money I had collected, I thought of my family. I said to myself, I have to send this amount of money to my family so they can pay for my loan from the moneychanger.

At the end of the day, the lady employer said, "Amanda, whatever money you collected, keep it, and maybe next week I'll bring you all to the supermarket together with Mary so you can buy something for yourself, and maybe you will also want to send a box to your family. You can buy something for them." I was smiling and extremely happy. At last, I can send gifts to my family for the first time. For sure, my parents will love it.

Chapter 28:
Visiting the Mall

After Ramadan, the lady's employer took us to the mall with Mary and the other helpers. The lady employer warned us not to talk to anyone, including other Filipinos. When the driver picked us up, I just enjoyed myself staring outside the car window because we couldn't even chitchat in the car. When we reached the Carrefour supermarket, we each took our own cart. The lady employer and Cindy were like two bodyguards. They made sure we didn't talk to anyone. We bought things for our families like body soap, noodles, canned food, and clothes. I bought 100 can goods and three boxes of unhealthy instant noodles - as we all know, noodles are easy to cook.

Most of the workers in the mall were Filipinos. One Filipino guy tried to talk to us, and a helper named Lina, who was with us, accidentally asked where the sugar was. The lady's employer immediately wanted to know what she said to the guy. She got really mad at Lina. She said, "I already warned you not to talk to anyone, and now you're disobeying and disrespecting us? We brought you here to buy your stuff – not to talk to anyone! It's dangerous! You have to respect our rules and regulations, you understand? You are in Saudi Arabia, not in the Philippines!" The Filipina helper apologized. I just kept quiet and stayed obedient.

I was so excited to see outside of Saudi Arabia. Date trees were everywhere; there are nice flowers along the streets and high buildings made of glass. Saudi Arabia is a very quiet place. You don't see many people walking around, especially women. In Dubai, there are many people walking in the streets. I remember when the male employer drove us to his parent's house, he saw a teenage female standing at the gate, pressing the doorbell of her house. He stopped driving until the teenager went in. He said, "Oh, no! Why did the parents allow her outside alone? It's dangerous!" Then the lady employer explained to me, "In Saudi Arabia, ladies can't walk alone outside. Why? They will end up in danger."

We bought many things for our families and for ourselves. But you know what? All the foods that I bought were really unhealthy. Back then, I didn't focus much on healthy eating. I liked eating canned foods and instant noodles because they are tasty. In the next chapter, I'll be sharing when and why I was hospitalized and got operated on because of sinus problems. These were all related to my bad food intake. It's important to choose healthy food to eat. I was naive and a bit ignorant, then. There were no books to read about a healthy lifestyle, and we didn't have cell phones or access to television for information.

While we were on our way home, it reminded me how poor we are in the Philippines, but seeing the outside of Saudi Arabia can be scary because of what the lady employer said. "You can't walk alone, or else you'll be raped or thrown in the desert." It was so unlike our place in the province, where you'll be safe even you walk in the middle of the night enjoying the bird's song and other sounds from nature. My life in Saudi Arabia was a challenging one; I never felt good since the people surrounding me aren't the type of people with whom I wanted to work. While it was true, there were many helpers there from my own country, the attitudes they seemed to develop with their positions were affecting my soul. But I am still grateful that I had the opportunity to experience and explore outside the Philippines.

At last, we reached home; I kept to myself while we were inside the car. The drive was boring! Even though it was only once in a while that I could see Mary, we still didn't talk much. Life is full of surprises. If you can't inspire or motivate yourself, you will end up depressed.

I was excited to check all the stuff we bought. I got lots of those tasty, unhealthy noodles with different flavors, soap for my family, coffee, new clothes, and slippers for my daughter and for myself.

The lady employer asked, "Amanda, how was your first experience shopping with us? Did you enjoy it?" I replied, "It was extremely exciting, Ma'am! Thank you so much for bringing us to the shop. I am so excited to surprise my family. It will be the first time they have ever received a big box from overseas." Then she said, "Seriously ... it's their first time to receive items from overseas? Don't you worry! Let's make your family happy this coming Christmas! I'll buy some things for your daughters!" Then she asked how old they were. That was the only time I had a real conversation with my lady employer. It was nice to get to know her a little better. She was kind of sweet, even if she wasn't mature enough to manage a family.

Chapter 29:
Life Goes On

I quickly prepared her lunch. After we had our lunch, I continued cleaning their big house. I also went to Cindy's house to cook for her and her husband. I remember when Cindy asked me to clean the master bedroom. Then she said, "Amanda, Sir is here. Don't come in!" She was very serious, and I ran quickly to the bathroom until I heard her laughing. "Amanda, I was just kidding!"

I was extremely nervous and scared, but she made me smile that day. "Sir is at work, Amanda!" We were laughing out loud. This couple didn't have a child yet. She liked baking and cooking, but I can't imagine washing all their dishes.

Every day was a tiring day for me. There were times I really felt I was going to collapse, especially when I smelled the dust. That night my head seemed like it was going to explode. I had a terrible headache, blocked nose, no appetite, and no energy to work anymore. I told the lady employer. She gave me a Panadol. I swallowed the Panadol, but I was getting worse. I took a cold shower to try and make the heat from my body go away. I wanted to vomit that night. I didn't sleep well but tried so hard.

The next day when I woke up, the headache was worse. I told the lady employer that I couldn't stand it anymore, so they made arrangements for me to see a doctor. The male employer dropped me off at the clinic, where there was lots of Filipino staff. They checked on my blood pressure, urine, temperature, etc. My nose was blocked, so I couldn't breathe very well. There the doctor found out I had sinusitis. I had an allergy to dust. The doctor prescribed many medicines. Actually, I hate taking medicines. I shared about my terrible experiences when I was 18. I took so many medicines that my body got tired of swallowing those capsules.

The doctor advised me to wear a mask every time I cleaned dusty areas. The male employer patiently waited for me. He paid for the bill, and we went back home. I thanked him, and I apologized for him having to spend money on me that day. When we reached home, the lady's employer explained to me how to take the medicines, although the doctor already explained everything to me. Then she reminded me how expensive the bill was. I replied, "I am aware, Ma'am. Thank you so much for your kindness."

I started cleaning again, even though I still wasn't feeling well. That day, I was thinking about my family and missing them so much. I reminded myself that if I didn't continue working, then I would not be able to keep my promise to my parents and my family. How would I support my family if I give up? What will happen to my dreams if I give up? I cried while I looked back at my regrets in life. I looked down on myself because I really didn't like this kind of job. This job isn't what I wanted in life. Since I was in the Philippines, I had been working as a helper. It's tiring, honestly, but I didn't have a choice. Sometimes I couldn't control myself and blamed everything on my parents. I am just honest here, but when I am feeling okay, I regret blaming them.

I remember when my mom told me, "I don't want you to experience what I experienced. That's why I kept telling you about my past." And my mom added, "I thought you learned from my past and from my story."

Chapter 30:
The Hardships

I only understood everything when I got married and had my own family - the hardships, trials, and regrets that I experienced during my married life. But what was done can't be undone. I have two beautiful daughters who inspire me every single day, and I want to work hard for them.

Every single day I had to be patient and work hard. Can you imagine yourself cleaning two four-story buildings with two cars, two gardens, two wide garages, two wide kitchens, and feeding two families every day without days off? Sometimes, employers brought me to other houses to work, as if I was a horse or a robot. If you looked at my fingers today, you would see all of the scars and cuts from cooking, cutting, harsh detergents, the weather – and too much hard work.

I bought notepads and pens when we went to get the groceries for whenever I had time to write. I just kept writing and writing without analyzing what I was writing about. Sometimes I wrote diaries, and sometimes I wrote long letters to my family. When I finished writing a letter, I asked the lady employer if I could send it and asked permission for their address. The lady's employer told me they didn't have an address yet since they were new to this house. I thought, "What? Of course, they had an address." I found out they don't give their address to anyone. She told me to pass my letter to Mary. Actually, I knew their address since I saw it in my documents when I applied, but I kept quiet and didn't say anything. I just asked the lady's employer to send it on my behalf.

Chapter 31:
The First Time I Saw Oprah

The lady employer and Cindy like to party a lot. So, at least three times a week, the couple let me take care of their daughter, and they let me watch TV with their daughter — but I wasn't allowed to change the channel. One night, it so happened that I tuned into one television show called "Dr. Oz," and the person he was talking with was Oprah Winfrey. I was touched by her talk. I can't remember what they were discussing, but I did remember her name. OPRAH WINFREY.

In that program, she spoke about charity. I was in tears listening to her talk. She was sitting on a couch facing Dr. Oz. She had curly thick hair, and she was wearing a red dress. I didn't get the address for sending mail since the employers came back from the party. It was 1:30 a.m. I was expecting to get another chance to watch Dr. Oz and Oprah talk on the same program later.

That morning, I quickly took out my notebook and pen and happily wrote Oprah Winfrey's name so I would not forget it. I lay down on my bed and kept thinking about what I'd watched and heard. I wanted to start writing, but I was tired the whole day and working till 1:30 a.m. You know the feeling when you are tired, and you want to relax, but you can't do it? I had to get up at 5:30 a.m., and I was tired. I almost wanted to give up, but what I heard from Oprah Winfrey inspired me. From that day on, I started gaining strength from within me. I slept and looked forward to seeing a brighter future for myself and for my family.

Chapter 32: Employer's Holiday After Ramadan

Once Ramadan was over, the whole family booked tickets to go on holiday. The lady's employer informed me one week ahead of time. Helpers cannot stay in the homes without their employers and must stay somewhere else, usually staying in their employer's parents' homes together with the rest of the helpers. I packed my things earlier that day. They were going on holiday for at least two weeks. I helped the lady employer pack all their stuff. While we were packing, she warned me not to talk too much with other helpers, to make sure I help with the household chores and washing cars, and to learn new recipes from other helpers. Before they dropped me off at the male employer's parents' home, they wanted me to clean the whole house, including Cindy's. That night they ordered McDonald's — and every time they ordered, they chose the big sizes.

Since I started eating fast foods and drinking Sprite, Coca-Cola, and 7-Up, I noticed my body becoming heavy. I was chubby, and my face was getting around, too. Every time someone saw me, they kept teasing me about eating so much. I remember one of the ladies' sisters told me, "Amanda, look at how you have changed! When I first saw you, you were so thin, but look how much weight you gained! It means you have a good life and good food to eat in my sister's kitchen. You eat too much, maybe?" I responded that the foods in Saudi Arabia were different for me. In my hometown, we didn't eat many processed foods because we had fresh fruits and vegetables from our farm. I didn't have the opportunity to drink anything like Coca-Cola or Sprite. I felt insulted when people kept telling me that I gained weight from eating too much. I didn't like my body overweight, but I do look beautiful with a chubby face (smiling).

The next morning, I woke up at 4:30 a.m. and quickly showered with cold water. I always showered because I didn't get a chance during the day since I had to sit with their daughter from morning to evening. If I moved slowly, then I would work till 3:00 a.m. Luckily, I am energetic and finished all the work on time, but I tell you - I worked like a robot with shivering legs and sweat dripping all over my body.

Thinking back, I wonder how I managed to stay with them for more than three years. Maybe the answer was "due to difficulties in the Philippines ... I didn't have a choice other than to work really hard." It is wonderful that I had to endure so many pains and hardships in life since I was a child. What a wonderful challenge for life! I had been dreaming of having a great job like others, but I felt I didn't have the power. I questioned myself while I was cleaning. Was this the job I deserved?

Then suddenly, Oprah Winfrey flashed in my mind. If she struggled a lot during her childhood and she became successful now, why can't I? She became my inspiration; whenever I felt low, I just pronounced her name clearly. I don't know why I admired her so much during my hard times. Every night, I prayed to Almighty God that He would send me someone to save my life - I meant a person who would become the instrument that would help me make my life change.

How would you feel if you kept working and working without communication with your loved ones? There were days I wanted to listen to my daughters' voices, to ask them how their day was, to watch how my parents fed my kids while I am away. These thoughts made me emotional. I felt sad because I didn't see my kids for many years. Until now, I was away from them, busily earning cash to support my family. I am happy and grateful for everything.

The couple dropped me off at their parents' home. I was to stay there for two weeks while they were on holiday. I had met the Filipina old Aunty, her name is Anna, and she is around 54 years old. She did not look friendly, but I smiled and introduced myself. She looked tired and haggard when I first saw her. She was brushing the kitchen floor when I arrived. She took me to her room so I could put away my things. When we went back down, she commanded me like a boss. I remember what she said: "There is a camera in this house, so you can't play and chat; you have to clean and be cooperative." I responded, "Yes. Don't worry; I'll help you clean; just let me know where I can find all the cleaning stuff." The truth was there was no camera. She was trying to scare us so we wouldn't be chatting all the time. Mary was also with us since the parents of her lady employer also went on a holiday to London.

Ana's employer's house had two kitchens and three cars. Oh, my God! Their house was bigger than a normal church in the Philippines with wide rooms, a wide living room, and three guest rooms for men and women. On the first day of the stay, she asked me to clean the master kitchen, clean all the cupboards, wipe all the utensils, brush the floors, and many other chores. Houses in Saudi Arabia are big and wide.

I couldn't imagine why there was only one helper in this big house. No wonder I saw spider webs and many dirty things — she can't clean everything! When I opened the fridge, every corner, both outside and inside, was extremely dirty. It was horrible! I cleaned the kitchen alone for more than three hours. Ana was lucky to have two extra helpers these two weeks because, for the first time, the whole house was getting clean.

I will always be an obedient person, and I learned to keep to myself since I don't want any arguments. I knew that these helpers weren't friendly — it was obvious through their actions and the way they talked. I pretended to be dumb. Seriously, I would rather be alone than with someone who doesn't know how to be a friend. I was so hungry and sweaty but so busy that I couldn't even cook my own noodles. Mary was busy cleaning the guest's rooms and toilets while the helper who stayed in this house for nine years was busy cooking and wrapping samosa.

Finally, it was lunchtime, and we ate lamb meat with tomato sauce and rice. Finally, we got a chance to talk to each other. But we had to eat fast because we still needed to finish our cleaning session by 7:00 p.m. It was going to be just the three of us staying in that big house for two weeks. After 15 minutes, no one touched the plates, so I stood up and started washing the dishes. Nothing would get done if these two helpers kept rolling their eyes. I pretended to be happy even when I was not. They are in their fifties, and I was only 25.

We continued our work while Ana was busy removing all the stuff from the cupboards. Then Mary said, "Why are you making us clean all the mess?" They started arguing, and I just kept quiet and busy doing my work. Isn't it nice when we have good communication and help each other? I couldn't lecture these two women. At their age, they should have known what they were supposed to do and not do.

At last! It was night time, time to rest. I'd been waiting for this time, so I could relax my feet since I had been standing from 5:00 a.m. to 7:00 p.m. We stayed in one room since the room was wide and big. We talked, but not too long. We laid our mattresses on the floor and set our own alarm clocks. I brought my own alarm. I showered, dried my hair, and then went to sleep. The next day, we had a good breakfast, and finally, Ana spoke to us nicely. She even smiled and talked about her family. It's a good feeling when every one of us starts our day with smiles on our faces. She asked us nicely to help her clean the whole house.

On the third day, we focused more on wrapping samosas and cooking different Arabic foods. The foods we prepared would be good for two months if maintained and kept in the freezer. I made notes of all the ingredients. Learning different kinds of recipes made me confused at the beginning. Every night I copied recipes from her recipe book until all the pages of my notebook were filled with recipes and tips.

On the fourth day, we washed the three cars, the wide playground, and the rooftop. We helped each other. After one week of stay, I learned a lot from

Ana, and of course, she got a lot of help from Mary and me. All of the corners in the house were shiny, clean, and fresh. We had another two days to stay. There were a few date trees in the backyard, and we harvested dates. It was fun harvesting dates, and we ate so many of them.

After two weeks, it was time to go back to a normal life of being alone when both of our employers got back from holiday. Mary and I said goodbye to each other and thanked Ana, and she thanked us too and gave us both hugs. She also gave us her address in the Philippines since we didn't have mobile phones at that time.

Chapter 33:
Shoes

My employers picked me up around six in the evening. The first thing my lady employer asked me was if I learned how to cook from Ana. I responded to her, "Yes, Ma'am, I have a long list." Once we reached home, I quickly showered their daughter, unpacked their luggage, and cooked dinner. They got me a souvenir from London - a nice pair of shoes. In my head, I exclaimed, "Wow! I have shoes to wear!"

I cleaned that night until 11:00 in the evening; the house was so dusty because it had been empty. I played with their daughter, then washed dishes and laundry. I went up to my room near midnight, very tired. It was almost 1:00 a.m. before I got to bed because I needed to shower and unpack my things. It would have been nice to look outside before I fell asleep, but my room didn't have a window.

My daily routine was always the same. The biggest thing that I was not happy about was that I was serving two families. I couldn't complain – and even if I wanted to, I had no one to complain to without a phone. I knew that no matter how tired I was, I was still able to survive, and as long as they didn't hurt me, everything would be all right. I was the happiest person when I overcame all the struggles and challenges.

The next day, the lady employer dropped me off with their daughter at their parents' home. There were other children present. They were playing, and I was watching them. The daughter of my employer was one year, five months at that time. She was a very active girl, very naughty, and she likes climbing everywhere.

I was so shocked when she accidentally knocked her head on the corner of a table and got injured. She was bleeding and cried until she turned purple. The cut was very deep, on her eyebrow close to her eye. I was so nervous and scared at that time. Then the grandmother quickly came down and took her granddaughter, and she scolded me non-stop. She said, "You didn't come here to gossip or whatever!"

To be honest, I was watching and following the baby girl wherever she went; it was an accident, and accidents happen. I apologized many times, but she ignored me. When the employer came, she was very mad at me. I waited for her to calm down before I explained what happened exactly. But sadly, she didn't accept my apologies that day. When we got home, she continued to scold me as if I was a killer.

I do understand; as a mother, we don't want our kids to be hurt. She didn't talk to me for a few days. I couldn't put my mind at ease, so I went out of my way to take good care of their child and cook her favorite lunch and prepare her favorite snacks. Even when I greeted her, she ignored me. At last, she spoke to me after the fourth day - what a relief.

Finally, I was able to start packing my things – over a year had passed, and I was going to see my family! I was excited!

Chapter 34:
Two Month Vacation

When you work away from your home and family, this is something you don't want to miss; it was the time most of the Foreign Domestic Workers waited for and looked forward to all year. I was never so happy to pack my things. In less than two years of working as a helper, I managed to buy land close to the city near my parents. They were very happy, especially my Dad, that I invested in something that was very valuable. I didn't have any savings yet since I sent all of my salaries to my family.

My kid's father didn't have a stable job and was struggling to overcome his health problems. In short, I became a mother and the father of my kids. I couldn't blame him if his health wasn't stable. My family had noticed something weird in him with the way he talked and through his movement. They didn't ask for support from him. He was suffering from some kind of mental illness, and it was very painful to see him that way. I really felt bad as I do care for him. The problem was, I couldn't even help him to go for check-ups because I needed to support our two kids. My salary was not always enough for their allowance (my salary was only $USD 150). When I heard the news that he was sick, I couldn't believe it at first. I was already depressed and stressed, and now a sickness was attacking him. I began hoping for him to regain his health.

One night before I left, the employer surprised me. She bought bags, shoes, clothes, and chocolates for my children. She treated me well because she wanted me to come back after two months of holiday. I knew my job was tough; however, I had to renew because I needed a job and salary. Back then, I was still innocent and very naive. I was scared to try new things, like applying to work in another country. People always told me that Saudi Arabia is one of the scariest countries in the world. The employer treated me well - not excellent, but the important thing was that I ate three times a day, and they didn't hurt me physically. I needed money badly for my family. I have a mission to accomplish because I promised myself I would take care of my family.

I still had a few days more before I was to leave, so I kept myself busy cleaning, ironing, and cooking and freezing enough food to last two months for their maintenance. It was a tiring time for a helper like me, but I motivated myself during that time. I told myself,

"Be patient, Amanda. You will see your family in a few days."

Most of my nights were sleepless since the lady employer loved to party almost every night together with Cindy. Sometimes they partied in their house. I had to prepare different kinds of dishes, sweets, and salads. They loved to drink lots of tea.

On my last day, I went to the other house to clean. All of their rooms, the bathrooms, guest rooms, and kitchen were very dirty and dusty - especially the curtains. At around 4:00 in the afternoon, the couple dropped me at the airport. Before I left, the lady employer gave me a gift: a gold necklace with a heart pendant. It was beautiful, and I'll be honest, it was my very first time receiving a gift – can you imagine how I felt? It was an amazing feeling.

Before I left, I changed into a t-shirt and a pair of jeans. OMG! I gained so much weight that I almost couldn't close the button of the 36-inch waistline jeans that I bought when we went to the market. For sure, all of the people in the Philippines were going to think I had a good life. Some people's perspective is always like that; if they see you are fat, they believe you are consuming expensive foods and live a good life. I used to think that way, too.

My employers went through my luggage before I left the house. I respect them as I stayed in their house for more than two years and three months, so it was their right to make sure none of their belongings had disappeared. I just waited with a big smile on my face because I was so excited to be seeing my family and hometown again.

The employer didn't make me wear the abaya or cover my face. I was so excited to get to the airport. My heart was beating so fast, and my excitement showed on my face. They drove me to the airport, and while we were on our way, the lady kept saying, "Please say hi to your kids and family. Take care of yourself, and don't forget to call us once you reach home." She handed me their home line and her mobile numbers.

It took about 30 minutes to reach the airport. The lady employer stayed in the car while the male employer brought me all the way inside the airport until I went inside the departure area. They were both very nice to me that day. The male employer patiently waited for almost two hours due to the long queue. Finally, we said goodbye to each other. As usual, I am the most obedient person you will ever know. I kept quiet in a corner while waiting for our plane. I didn't talk to anyone because most of the people were from Sri Lanka. I did walk around to explore what they called duty-free and to see the beauty of the surroundings. Only when I went inside the plane did I meet a few Filipinos.

Chapter 35:
The Long Flight Home

I was embarrassed to let people see my hands because they were so dry and scarred. It wasn't until we were about to eat our lunch that the lady beside me noticed my fingers. She then started to talk to me. She was working as a nurse, so her fingers were nice and clean. She gave me one small container of Vaseline. She advised me to put the cream on during night time. I was very grateful to that lady. Actually, I bought a big container of Vaseline later, and I applied it at night as she said, but it didn't work.

We began talking. She started telling me how many helpers got abused by their employers. She had a nice smartphone and showed me the news of abuse. Some helpers were raped, thrown through windows, kicked, punched in their faces, or some parts of their body. Some helpers were locked in a room without food or water, and some were killed. Lots of helpers were not fed well, and they became very skinny and bony. She showed me all the pictures that were posted in a group on Facebook

– I didn't know anything about Facebook or social media because I didn't have a phone.

Then she asked me how my experience was with my Saudi employers. I told her that my employers were kind and never hurt me physically. I was fed three times a day. It did not matter how hard I worked because they treated me well; that's why I accepted the second contract. I added that my employers were both young – eight years younger than I was. Sometimes they did scold me because of mistakes I made, but that was normal. She smiled and congratulated me; however, she felt bad about my ugly fingers.

We had a connecting flight from Saudi Arabia to Riyadh. The lady that was beside me had a different seat, so I didn't see her anymore. At Dubai Airport, I met many Filipino, and I enjoyed chatting with them. Most of them were helpers, and we're talking mostly about their experiences. Some of them were dressed very simply like me, some were wearing thick jewelry and dressed up nicely, and some looked very elegant. Then I looked at myself, very chubby with a big belly and big arms but still looking good.

Non-stop flight time from Manila to Riyadh is around 11 hours 15 minutes. The average flight between Manila and Riyadh takes close to 13 hours. However, some airlines could take as long as 37 hours based on the stopover destination and waiting duration. I was flying on Emirates Airlines. Before I went on the plane, I approached one of the Filipina women to text my family and let them know I'll be arriving in 11 hours 30 minutes. My Mom, Thomas, and Jim were going to fetch me at the airport. They were excited.

The moment we went on the plane, the flight attendant gave us all pieces of paper for us to fill out some information. I didn't have a pen – almost none of us did – and everybody was passing and borrowing pens to and from each other. I waited for my seatmate to finish, and then I borrowed her pen. It was funny because most of us couldn't even answer all the simple questionnaires. This was the problem that I observed; if you were working and focusing on your work of being a helper, you did not have the opportunity to learn other things! Most of us had trouble with spelling. The flight attendants and crew had to help us explain what certain words meant! I wasn't even able to answer all the questions. But I looked at my seat mate's answers and got some idea. With no books, no TV, no newspapers, and no cell phone, my mind was stuck.

For two years, all I had been able to do was focus on cleaning, cooking, ironing, cleaning cars, and taking care of a baby. I'm telling you, even though I finished a degree, since I didn't apply what I learned, didn't continue reading, writing, and socializing with other people, my mind became rusty. In Saudi Arabia, in 2006, you were lucky if you had books to read or a mobile phone while you were working as a helper. I will tell you the big difference later in the next chapter when I worked in Singapore, how socializing, surrounding myself with books, and having a cell phone affected my thinking. It will be a very interesting part of my story. Keep reading until the end; I assure you – you will learn something that you can apply to your own life and make a difference. I am trying to tell you everything in detail, so you know exactly how I overcame all these struggles in my life.

When everybody finished filling out the forms, we handed them to the crew and fastened our seatbelts. Oh, my God! Another funny observation: if you aren't a traveler, you don't know how to fasten a seatbelt, even if the crew already explained how to do so! What you have to do is to observe other people doing it – but you will still get confused! I was like that then – but not anymore!

Our plane started to fly from Dubai to the Philippines. Woohoo! In about 12 hours, I would finally see the Philippines! Some of the passengers on the plane were from other countries like Japan, Israel, Canada, Spain, and many other countries. Some people traveled to the Philippines for a holiday. After the plane took off, most of the people chose to sleep. Some were talking, and some were reading books or magazines. I was seated near a window, so I watched the clouds for about an hour and then tried to sleep.

I got two meals on the plane. Before the male employer handed me my plane ticket, he told me, "Amanda, I ordered you expensive meals so you won't be hungry before landing in the Philippines." I enjoyed my meals very much.

After long hours on the plane, we were about to land at the airport. I noticed from the window how amazing the clouds were. When I first traveled, I sat in the middle, and I wasn't that comfortable. I observed that having window seats is much more entertaining. I enjoyed both the view and the experience. When you travel during the day, you'll get to admire the scenery of clouds and landscapes. Sitting by the window allows you to feel separate from other passengers, too. I loved the views from plane windows. Where else do you get an opportunity to see the world from that vantage point and see the beauty of the earth and the sky? I still get excited seeing changes in geography, seeing snow-capped mountains rising from a green plain, and then suddenly seeing the different shades of water in the oceans. Even clouds can be exciting. I wished I had a camera so I could capture the view, but I didn't have one at the time.

Everybody was smiling and so excited to hug and see their families. When our plane landed, everyone was busy taking their things out from the overhead bins. Then we went out and collected our luggage. It took more than two hours of waiting for my luggage to come out. I couldn't wait to see my family, but I needed to be patient.

When you are walking through the airport, some of the staff thinks you are rich. A staff member offered to help me push my luggage, and I let him do the job since I had four suitcases – and I thought it was free, but after he dropped me off close to the waiting area, this guy tried to charge me a lot of money. I told him I thought it was part of his job to help; however, I gave him 150 pesos.

Chapter 36:
Seeing My Family
After Two Long Years

Thomas saw me first. We hugged each other. At first, they didn't recognize me, especially my mom. My mom hugged me with tears in her eyes. My family's first impressions were, "Wow! You are beautiful, white, and you look very healthy!" I was laughing at that because my mom called me very healthy when I had a big belly and big arms. Before they started carrying my luggage, they told me that they went to the airport to fetch me the day before, because the Philippines time is 4 hours ahead of Saudi Arabian time! We all laughed at that. It's part of the experience anyway, and it's more fun experiencing stupid things in life - sometimes so you can learn from it sometimes so you can just laugh. They went to the airport two times! My poor family! I didn't instruct them well enough.

We hired a cab, heading to our town's bus station. We talked excitedly, laughing together. I could tell how Mom had aged; her skin was so dark from being under the sun daily. I asked about my kids. I knew my Mom and Dad sacrificed so much taking care of them. I had only a little money. Seeing my Mom, Jim, and Thomas made me cry, and all the more, I wanted to pursue success and not have to see them experience many struggles. Deep inside, I was hurting to see them looking pitiful. My mom told me that the kids were growing so fast. They were very talkative and became a stress reliever. We reached the bus station. From there, it would be 9 hours before we get home.

I couldn't wait to see my children and the rest of the family. We brought some snacks so we can have something to eat on the bus. After seven hours of traveling, we were dropped off at the market. We bought groceries and planned to take a tricycle back home. We couldn't fit in one tricycle because I had four big bags, so we hired two. I was extremely tired after more than 20 hours of travel. After the tricycle dropped us off at the stop, we still needed to walk the last 30 minutes on the rocky and muddy path (I mentioned before that our house was located on a hillside, in a mountainous area). We reached our home at about 10:00 a.m., and there I saw my kids with dirty clothes and smiling happy faces. They were very happy when they saw me. I carried them, and the moment I saw them, I quickly showered them, changed them into new clothes that my employer bought for them. My kids were cute and had pretty faces once they were cleaned and dressed up.

I started opening my luggage so I could surprise my family with what I brought while my Dad and Mom were busy cooking our lunch. In my area, when someone comes back from visiting overseas, all the neighbors and relatives come to visit. We had a lot of visitors! I bought many chocolates and soap bars, and I distributed them like I was Santa Claus that day! Even the visitors benefitted — but, of course, this is our culture.

We believe that the more you give, the more blessings you receive.

My kids, nieces, and nephews were busy eating chocolates until all their faces, clothes, and fingers were covered in chocolate. It was fun watching these little kids and seeing how they enjoyed it. I gave my Mom and Dad their favorite flavored coffee and handed them cash. I saw how happy they were. I thanked them for taking care of my girls while I was away. That day, I called my lady employer to inform her that I arrived safe and sound and to tell her how grateful and excited my family was when I handed them the things she had bought for them. We had our lunch together with family and neighbors.

I noticed our house was the same, with no improvements made since I left. I also saw that some of the wood was broken and had holes from ants. I couldn't put my mind at ease; deep inside, my heart hurt seeing my family in this state. My mind was spinning with dreams of having a nice house, so my family could have a safer place to stay. I thought back to when I was typing outside my employer's condominium with tears in my eyes. I thought that working overseas for more than two years would solve all our problems and fix our poor house. I dreamed it was being fixed, but it didn't happen. I thought I would be able to give my family a better life.

Our house was very messy and dirty; I didn't complain because I understood how busy my parents were. If you saw my house, you'd know you wouldn't be able to sleep there, with many mosquitoes all day and all night. No matter how poor and tough our life was, we managed to laugh and smile. We still didn't have electricity. One of our neighbors, about 10 minutes away from our home, managed to install electricity through the help of their sister, who was working in America. They are the only family in our area who managed to get electricity. Most of the people thought they were rich because of it. It cost a large amount of money since the main source was very far away.

I told my family that one day we would have electricity, too, but we would have to build our house close to the city. I have a lot of dreams in life, especially how I could improve our lives. But it isn't easy for me because I am alone earning a living. I'm aware that I'm not just helping my kids; I am helping support my parents and my two sisters, and I am the main person who provides everything. Even though my parents were selling fruits and vegetables, it did not bring in that much. I reminded myself.

"If others can do this, I can, too. I need patience, perseverance, and sacrifice."

After two days of vacation, I brought my family to the city and let them buy the things they needed for school. We bought only the necessary stuff as they knew I had only a little money left. I treat them to a fast-food restaurant called "Jollibee" so they can also experience eating in a nice restaurant. I also wanted my little girls to experience new surroundings and to begin socializing with different people because our place in the mountains was rather isolated. I didn't eat much since I had already eaten so much fast food in Saudi Arabia.

My money was gone after one week at home. I had found myself feeding the relatives and neighbors that visited me every day. Because people in the Philippines think working overseas makes you rich, you can't be rude and tell them, "I'm sorry, we have to eat our breakfasts, lunches, and dinners, and we don't have enough to share with you." I called my employer and begged her to let me go back without finishing the two months holiday. She laughed at me, and she said, "I thought you missed your family badly!" I told her, "Yes, I do miss them badly, but I can't endure seeing them without proper food." Then the lady employer told me I had to stay because when I went back, I would have to stay another two years before I could see my family again.

I stayed for two months. I cleaned the house and took care of my kids while my parents were busy planting vegetables and making charcoal. Our life was back to normal – the normal before I had any money. It rained a lot during my vacation, and mud was all over the place. The bad thing about our area was that in heavy rain the drinking water from the river turns brown, so we would have to walk to other places further away to get some clear water to drink. You might have to walk at least 15-20 minutes away. I didn't want to add stress to my parents, so I did the job when it was needed. I took a big gallon jug and filled it with water. I had to carry all the way back. It was heavy, and I walked barefoot. The road was very rough in zigzag directions and very muddy. I made that trip at least three times because I wanted our big pail to be filled with clean water.

I did buy a Nokia phone to receive calls and texts. I received many calls from friends, and sometimes I talked so much during the day that Mom gave me a nickname: 'Broadcaster.' My Mom said she enjoyed my company since the house was filled with a lovely loud voice produced by me! One day before my last week, Mom and I had a long discussion. We discussed how we could save money to start building our new house since I already bought the land. My salary is difficult to budget. I hadn't started working again yet, but we borrowed some money from the moneylender in our town at 10% interest.

Chapter 37:
My Letter to Oprah Goes Up in Smoke

I wrote almost ten pages to Oprah Winfrey while I was in Saudi Arabia. I told myself that once I reached home in the Philippines, I would like to find her address, but I didn't have the chance to find it since we didn't have television or the internet. We were using firewood for cooking our food. One day was raining so heavily that my mom took a paper to get the fire going on the wet wood – and she accidentally grabbed my letter that I was supposed to send to Oprah Winfrey. It was kind of old and a bit crumpled. It was dark, so my mom didn't notice.

The next morning, I was looking for a paper to rewrite the letter to make it neater. My plan had been to let my mom keep the letter for me, so when any one of our family members finds Oprah's address, then they can send it on my behalf. I know my mom still remembers this story. She told me, "You are crazy to do such things!" I smiled back and said, "You never know! Maybe Oprah will have time to read my story." But sadly, my long letter was now ash. I couldn't scold my mom. I spent so much time writing that letter. I talked to my Mom about Oprah Winfrey and how she helped poor people, and I thought of trying to send my letter to her - not to ask for money, but to let her know how much she inspired me during my hard time. Again, my mom laughed at me and discouraged me from doing such things.

I started packing my things before my last two days to be with my family. I had to travel to Manila at least one day earlier so I wouldn't miss the flight. It was a painful feeling leaving my family. I loved them so much, so I need to sacrifice for them. My Dad was so busy making charcoals, carrying heavy woods from far places. I didn't see my Dad relax at all in the entire two months of my vacation. He was busy all the time. It was painful to watch him walking with one amputated leg. He smoked a lot and was still a heavy coffee drinker. He was also skinny. I suspected before he had been suffering from diseases, but we never had extra money to send him to see a doctor. Sigh! Our life was pitiful and poor. I wanted to do something for them, and that's why I needed to return to Saudi Arabia. My Dad's simple request was to have a Carabao to make it easier for him to collect big branches of wood. I promised to buy him one. I loved the big smile on his skinny, bony face.

I never wanted my kids to see me leave. I left early in the morning, and I told my kids I'll go to the market and buy them good toys and snacks. I didn't hug my mom. I was a bit shy about it, but I secretly left a long letter under her pillow. I expressed everything there - my plans, my dreams, how grateful I am that they took good care of my kids. I knew that once my mom read my letter, she would be in tears. My mom also was very grateful because I am the only child who is willing to help them.

Three minutes away from home, I heard the loud cries of my oldest daughter, then five years old. I did not want to leave them! Especially after seeing my youngest daughter — she's very skinny and looks malnourished. My parents told me that mostly they eat rice and they just have to pour with hot coffee or sometimes oil with soya sauce. My heart broke when I heard those stories. I want to do something for them — that's why I have to leave them and work overseas. I need to get them out of that unhealthy environment with all the charcoal smoke.

To all the Mothers who are lucky to have a responsible husband, a treasure that! Love your husband back. I can't blame my husband right now since he's suffering from his own health problems. We parents have the responsibility to take good care of our kids. Give all your best to support them, but don't forget to take care of yourself so you can continue to give the best of yourself to others. I may not be the luckiest woman in terms of marriage, but I tell you — I am lucky to have beautiful kids. Forgive me for mentioning my kids' Dad; some people may hate me for leaving him, but I have to be honest here. However, I do care for him, and I'll help him if I can.

While I was walking the rough road heading to the jeep's station, I kept imagining things; there were many things in my head. I tried not to cry anymore, but I couldn't stop, especially after hearing my daughter's voice calling me and screaming, "MAMA! MAMA! MAMA! Please come back!" My eyes were already swollen and very red, and I was wiping my nose over and over and sneezing. I took a deep breath before reaching the place where I was to pick up a tricycle or jeep—leaving my family to achieve a specific goal required immeasurable sacrifice. It was a painful feeling, but as a Mom with full responsibility, I had to endure everything, no matter how tough the job was.

I rode in a jeep, and it took 30 minutes before we reached the bus station heading to Manila City. There I waited about two hours before the bus came. Luckily there were few passengers this time, so I got the chance to sit and relax my back. It took us seven hours before we reached the city. I went straight to the agency, and I spoke to the owner. There I told everything! I asked the owner if he could talk to my employer to increase my salary because I am working for two families. I told the owner that the first agreement I made was for only one family, but when I reached the place, I served two. I told him how large their building was and how I only got 3-4 hours' sleep a night. The owner of the agency said he would talk to the male employer.

Once I collected all the documents, I went to the hotel and stayed for one night before heading to the airport. The next day, I went to the airport very early. I didn't have much strength, and I felt alone. It was all because I loved my family.

Chapter 38:

Back to Riyadh

I felt very sad and lonely at the airport. I wanted to talk to my family before getting on the plane. I didn't carry my phone with me because I am not allowed to use phones in Saudi Arabia. I wanted to use the telephone from the airport, but I didn't have any money at all. I let my emotions run through my body until I went inside the plane. I was sobbing. It was a painful feeling to be away from my family. I took a deep breath. The flight attendants all greeted us with beautiful smiles. I went to my designated seat, and there I relaxed my head and tried not to think of my family. I grabbed a copy of the magazine in front of me and focused on reading.

Finally, the plane took off. Everybody was quiet and sleeping, so I tried to close my eyes, but I wasn't able to sleep. My thoughts were with my family. I could imagine their faces and situations. I have to do something for these family members. Finally, after ten hours of long travel, we reached Riyadh. Like before, I waited for at least four hours before my employer picked me up at the airport. Both of the couples fetched me, and they were both excited to see me. While we were on our way to the house, I chatted non-stop with the lady employer. When we reached home, I quickly washed my hands and played with their child while they checked my stuff from the Philippines. They had to make sure I didn't bring a mobile phone with me or anything that is against their rules and regulations. I brought some cooked foods that can last for a month for Mary that her family wrapped.

I never rested, and instead, I started cleaning their house. It was extremely dusty and dirty all over the place. I was tired, hungry, and sleepy. This was the challenge most helpers need to overcome. Others can't take it because their bodies are weak. One has to drink lots of water and, of course, don't forget to talk to the employer. If your body can't take it anymore, you have to let them know you are hungry. If you don't talk, then how can they read what's on your mind? Not all employers had a good heart, so speak first. Don't starve to death. Sometimes employers thought you had a good time spending your holiday with your family. They have a good life, and they don't understand what you experienced. Be strong and learn how to talk nicely, and don't forget.

Before finishing the household chores, I asked the lady employer for permission to eat something, or else I'd be very weak working long hours. She let me stay in the kitchen until I finished eating some sandwiches. While the male employer was out for groceries, I quickly went out to clean the outside. I didn't use water as I needed only 30 minutes to clean. Oh, my God! If you can see how thick the dust was, you'd end up sneezing the whole time. I didn't have a mask yet at that time, so I had to endure inhaling the thick dust.

While I was in the Philippines, I went to see a Doctor from ENT since I always suffered from terrible headaches. The doctor found out I have sinusitis and needed urgent action. I am allergic to dust and get easily sick. There were cysts inside my nose that blocked me from breathing. I ignored it since I didn't have enough cash for the surgery. I had only medicines.

As usual, I did the same house cleaning, car washing, babysitting, ironing, and cooking for the two families. The lady employer let me use her phone, so I could let my family know I reached Saudi Arabia safely. She let me use only three minutes since calling from overseas was still expensive. I was grateful at least to hear my family's voices. I spoke to my mom and my daughters. They were so happy, and I promised them that once I received my salary, I'd send them so they could buy some nice clothes and nice food to eat. Then we said goodbye to each other.

When I heard my loved ones' voices, even from far away, I became more energetic; I could perform my job well, and I was inspired and motivated. My family's voices became my strength while I was away from them. I was lucky that my employers let me call them. There were some employers who wouldn't allow their maids to talk to their family the entire year. There were a lot of employers all over the world who were very mean to their helpers, but I still considered myself lucky because the employer that I worked with cared for me and would let me use their mobile phone to talk to my family once in a while - like once in six months or once a year.

Hopefully, soon, employers who treat their maids like strangers will realize that maids are human and have feelings, too. Some employers don't realize that maids aren't machines, and they work them like robots.

As maids, we do our part to serve employers to their satisfaction. We cook nice foods for them, clean their bathrooms, wash their bedsheets, iron their clothes, hand them water even though they have feet and hands to use, and serve many people in one house doing multiple tasks. They should appreciate all we do, even when we are far from our families. We want to be treated so we can deliver our best.

The next day, the lady employer brought me to her parents' home, so I can see Mary and give her the stuff from her family. There, I released all of my emotions. I just started working, and after two months of holiday, my thoughts were still with my family. I struggled at first, wondering how I could overcome homesickness. If I let myself be sad and dwell on the poor side, I would end up stressed and depressed. The best thing is to do something productive.

Thank goodness I had the chance to talk to Mary (although she's kind of strict). She fed me and let me eat as much as I could. I was skinny and old-looking again – that's the reality of staying in the Philippines without proper food and struggling to survive. It's a long journey to be poor; no matter how hard we work, we can't have a good life. The good life I was dreaming of - to be together with my family, working together and helping each other, being able to travel with my family, able to save money for the future – would take me many years to achieve since I am the only member of our family who is earning a paycheck monthly.

That's what happened to Mary; she had been working with the same employer for about twenty years but still the same, sole support and help for her family. She sacrificed so much that she forgot to enjoy her own life. She was dedicated to helping her family. I won't allow that to happen to me because I want my family to explore things. I am the only person who will take responsibility to teach them new things and not focus on staying in the forest forever. I had to be away from my family so I could build a house close to the city. Once they live in a better place with electricity, where they can see lots of neighbors, and surround themselves with good people, then they will be able to open their eyes to new opportunities.

We went back home after almost nine hours of stay. We had dinner, and I helped Mary clean the big house, as usual. The moment we reached home, I quickly went to Cindy's house together with the lady employer's daughter to do a quick dusting and to cook a simple dinner for the couple.

Then, Ramadan was almost around the corner, so everybody got busy bringing lamb meat into their houses, and I had to manage my time efficiently. It was a busy month for helpers.

Chapter 39:

Celebrating Ramadan

For The Third Time

Since I already knew what to do, and this was the third time, I celebrated Ramadan with these families. For me, Ramadan was the hardest part of being a maid. I was alone looking after two families with only two to three hours of sleep a night until the holiday ended. There were no breaks because I needed to prepare a complicated meal. However, I overcame all these difficulties and hard times. The only things that I couldn't stand were my migraine headaches. Even though I took medication, I suffered heavily. The more I swallowed a pill, the more I felt like it was getting worse. There was a time my nose bled from the extreme dust and hot weather.

Even if when I dusted and cleaned every day, if the sandstorm attacked, it wasn't enough! It was extremely hot, and there was no fan in the kitchen. When I got up in the morning, I felt exhausted because I wasn't sleeping well. I told the lady employer, and all she could do was offer me more Panadol. I was tired of taking it because it didn't have any effect.

The lady employer reminded me that during the month of Ramadhan, Muslims must refrain from eating, drinking, smoking, marital relations, or getting angry during the daylight hours. In addition, those fasting are supposed to refrain from bad habits and be more diligent in prayer and give to charities, as well. It is believed that fasting heightens spirituality and develops self-control.

While it is expected that people will keep to their normal activities during the fast, it should be needless to say that the lack of liquid and food during the day and the unusual sleep and meal schedule soon take their toll. We always expected many guests during the Ramadan family get-togethers. I remember once before Ramadan, I was harassed by one of the drivers. One evening, Cindy asked me to collect something outside of the driver. The driver grabbed my breast, and I kicked him. He quickly ran away. It's true what I heard from the lady employer and the lady on the plane it's dangerous to go out alone. You will be raped or killed because those men who don't have a wife will be lonely. I didn't tell anyone what had happened. I was nervous, and it was only the first time they asked me to collect a package, so I let it go.

One week before Ramadan, I was busy wrapping samosas like I did the last time. I wrapped more than a hundred and stored them in the freezer. I did the same for the other couple. I started working from 4:30 a.m. to almost 2:00 a.m. It was extremely tiring. I also mentioned before that I almost collapsed going up to my room since my body didn't have enough strength, and my feet were numb. It was the same this year. It had been a while since I had the chance to talk to my family.

Chapter 40:

My Mom's Mini

Grocery Store

Before I went to bed, I stood in front of the mirror and stared at myself. I didn't like what I saw in the mirror, again chubby and with a dull face. I wasn't allowed to use any beauty products except Dove soap.

There wasn't enough freedom when someone could go through all your stuff. Most of the people in the Philippines thought you had a good life working overseas! Some of my relatives would want to borrow money, and if I didn't lend it, they would gossip about me – some would even curse me. Our family experienced that. When some of our relatives heard the news that I was working overseas, they kept going back to our house, borrowing rice or groceries from my mom's mini grocery store.

I let my mom start a small business so they could help. These people promised to pay my mom back within three days to one week, but they would always disappear. I told my mom not to say hurtful words. I felt bad because my Mom and Dad carried all the heavy goods on their shoulders or head and would end up bankrupt. Many people took advantage of our kindness.

I remember since I was a child, my parents were both generous enough to try to feed everybody. They would make a way to prepare food for whoever visited simple food from our garden. My mom always reminded us to be nice to everyone, to be respectful and kind. Never answer back to adults and always be helpful. Mom always said, the more you give, the more blessings you receive. To this day, I carry all those good lessons that my mom taught us.

Chapter 41:

Summarizing Saudi Arabia

I'll try to summarize all my experiences in Saudi Arabia. After the celebrations of Ramadan, the whole family would leave for the holiday and be gone for at least 15 days. So, as usual, I had to stay at Mary's employer with Mary and Ana. It was just the three of us helpers there. We helped each other clean the entire big house. At least there, I went to sleep a little earlier and got up at 5:00 a.m.

During my stay, Mary gave me a hint that both of us would receive a Nokia phone from our employers when they came home from holiday. We were both happy and thinking in advance how we could buy top-ups (added cell phone credit), and laughed with all the excitement. For the first time, they were going to buy us phones after years of service, especially Mary, who'd been working there for more than ten years. The good news was that Cindy was planning to hire her own helper. Thank God!

After 15 days away, my employer picked me up. They brought presents for me from overseas. The lady employer asked me if I knew someone I could recommend to them as a helper – someone who was at least close to my family or relatives. They appreciated my work performance, so they wanted my recommendations rather than hiring a helper from the agency. They asked me to call my family and ask my mom If she knew some of our relatives who could work overseas. My mom quickly mentioned Laila from our village. The next morning, we called our mom to confirm whether Laila wants to work. Laila was extremely excited, and she said yes quickly. The lady's employer requested a video call, and I told her that Laila didn't speak English well, but she could work and follow instructions.

A week later, they set up a video call so that they could have a conversation before hiring her. Laila needed to go down to the city for the video call since she was also using a Nokia phone that didn't have internet. It was only then that the lady employer realized that we were a very poor family, and she asked many questions. "Amanda, how can you live without electricity? What light does your family use at night? How can they cook their food?" She asked many questions. I smiled and told her we survived like that for over 25 years. She couldn't believe it.

Chapter 42:

A Typhoon Hits

the Philippines

One night they were watching the news, and they quickly called me to watch with them. It was all about a strong typhoon. On the news, they showed all the houses filled with water and all the stuff that got flushed away by the strong winds and water. I told them that the Philippines always suffered, and we experienced terribly strong typhoons. Thousands of families are made homeless by the strong typhoon, and thousands of people would die from the floods.

My family had been lucky because we stayed in higher places in the mountains. The only things usually affected by strong typhoons were my parent's rice planting, fruits, and some of our trees. The lady employer commented that it was heartbreaking. But they would never offer any help, even though they are one of the richest families in the Kingdom – not that I was expecting them to. We were taught to be independent and not to ask for help from others.

Laila went to the city, and we video called her. Cindy confirmed her. We had to wait at least two months before she could reach Saudi Arabia because she needed to be processed. I am happy that, finally, Cindy will have her own helper – especially because she was pregnant.

At last, I got the phone already bought by the male employer, and he set it up. They asked me for at least five contact numbers to be added to the contacts, so I gave my Mother-in-law's phone number and my family's contact number. Then he made sure that I couldn't add any other contact numbers to the phone. Before they handed me the phone, they already told me I could not talk to anyone except for the contacts they added. I responded to them excitedly, and I said, "Yes, Ma'am." The lady employer handed me the phone. She was smiling and happy, too. I hugged her and said, "Thank you so much, Ma'am." I was so excited to touch the phone, but I had to wait for the night time since that day was a busy day for everybody. They had just returned from holiday, so I had to focus on looking after their daughter and cleaning the dirty clothes.

The day was over, and YES! It was nighttime, and I was finally able to touch my phone. I was smiling widely as I quickly dialed my family's mobile phone number. Even though it was late at night, I couldn't wait any longer. I knew it was late in the Philippines, but I was so excited. Seriously! I dialed two times, and no one answered my call. I was disappointed, but after five minutes I dialed again, and finally, my sister picked up the phone. It was 3:00 a.m., and everyone was still sleeping. I told them I was sorry about the time difference, but I was so excited to tell them the good news that my employer bought me a new phone. She quickly woke my mom up, who was excited to say hello to me, and then everybody got up, including my two daughters.

After 15 minutes of chatting, I didn't realize that I exceeded my limit! I had used up the entire top-up. After the call, I was nervous because the lady employer told me when she handed me the phone to be careful of my phone usage because a top-up is expensive. If I could not discipline my phone usage, they would deduct it from my salary. I ended up paying the top-up. I learned then to call if there's an important thing to say. It didn't matter; it was only my first time, and I learned quickly.

I slept with a smile on my face. The next morning, the lady employer asked me how I slept and did I manage to talk to my family. She checked my phone, and she was very disappointed when she found there was no remaining balance on my top up. I apologized, and she didn't top it up for me. So that was my experience. Lesson learned: learn how to value every little thing. Just because you are expecting a salary, it doesn't mean you should drain your hard-earned money.

Two months passed by, Laila processed all her documents, and plane tickets were sent to the agency. She was ready to fly. Mary's employer asked for another recommendation, so one of my classmates in university before, named Marivic, also came to Saudi Arabia. We become four helpers from the Philippines, and we were friends in the Philippines. When they reached Saudi Arabia, however, we couldn't see or talk to each other. We only had a chance to see each other when the family got together for Ramadan, family reunions, and when the lady employer dropped me off at her parent's home.

Chapter 43:
Dealing with Co-Helpers

When Laila and Marivic came, everything was okay at first. Since Marivic worked together with Mary, it meant there were two helpers in one big house. The one who stayed longer in that house was too strict, and she commanded like a boss. Since Laila was new to this kind of environment, she was still ignorant of how to use appliances like microwaves, washing machines, and others. When I went to their place, Marivic looked very tired, stressed, and unhappy. She didn't talk at our first meet up because she was scared to share with me what was happening.

I knew already what was going on since I worked with Mary before – I would stay with her when both our employers were on holiday, so I knew exactly how she treated others. While Mary was showering, we had the chance to talk to each other. Marivic said she couldn't stand her bossy attitude and the fact that she made her do most of the work. She said she would often go to bed crying because of Mary's hurtful words. She said that one afternoon she wanted to eat, but Mary stopped her, so she learned how to steal foods and eat in the bathroom. She said that Mary would call her slow and stupid if she didn't finish her work on time. Marivic said, "I need someone to talk to, and I have no one to share my sufferings with. I'm afraid I can't finish my contract, Amanda."

I advised her: "You have to be patient, do the things that your employer asks you to do. Do your responsibilities and never complain. Eat if you are hungry, and never answer her back since she's older than us. Talk to her in a calm and low voice." She was crying while telling me how she was treated by co-helpers. At least the employers are good to her. "When I spoke nicely to Mary, she wouldn't listen, and instead, she got so upset with me. The way she rolled her eyes! You could read everything. She hated us!"

I knew that jealousy was the main reason behind her attitude, but we still had to respect her. These things happened for months and years. In this case, I learned another lesson again. I started writing down in my diary notes whenever something happened to us - good or bad. When Laila also experienced the same treatment, I told her to be patient, too. It was hard to understand her attitude. The way she talked, her action towards us – she was very rude. I shared with Laila and Marivic about my first experiences with her.

At the end of the day, we managed to smile and laugh. Tips: don't focus on the negative side; focus on the good things she had done for us. And I told both of them, no matter how rude she was, we still owed her. We should be very grateful she had helped us to reached Saudi Arabia, or else we wouldn't be able to help our families.

We went back home with the lady employer together with Marivic. It's funny because we were not allowed to talk once our employers were with us. While we were inside the car, we pinched each other and smiled.

After a few months, Mary's employer hired another maid, and this time Mary's sister Susanne came. Now there were three helpers in that house. We thought that Mary could get along together with her sister. We were wrong. One day, the lady employer dropped me there with their daughter.

Mary's sister was crying while cleaning the stairs; I asked her why. She also shared with me how her sister treated her badly. She said, "It's tough to work with her. I would rather give up and go back to the Philippines than to argue with my own sister every single hour. My blood pressure goes up!" I thought she was kidding, but I heard with my own ears how Mary talked to her. My God!

One night, around 7:00 p.m., we were waiting for the lady employer to pick us up. Susanne was shivering, and her skin was very pale. I didn't have any idea about a person who suffered from high blood pressure. She collapsed, and I quickly called out to Mary. She was very cold, and she said her fingers were numb; I massaged her fingers. I saw how nervous Mary was when she saw Susanne shivering. She called their employer, and they quickly took her to the hospital. We were worried she wouldn't survive.

Since then, the other helper realized that due to her rudeness, attitude, and actions, she was hurting someone. After that incident, everything changed. Sometimes, you only change when something bad happens to others. Then you realize your mistakes. In life, you have to learn to love yourself first before you learn how to love and take care of others. We are all human beings; we have feelings, and we have our own thinking. Be good to others. I believe it will come back to you how you treated others.

I was alone one day, cleaning the whole house when suddenly someone called my mobile number. I thought it was a call from the Philippines. I didn't see the number. I was busy mopping the floor and very tired and very sweaty. I said hello, and the person on the other line didn't say anything, so I said once again, "Hello?" No one answered, so I hung up the phone. When the lady employer came back, she opened the door, and she was screaming loudly, "Amanda, Amanda, where are you? Come here!" She threw her bag in front of me. I was so nervous and scared, not knowing why she was screaming at me. I said, "Yes, ma'am, what happened?"

"Come here, show me your phone - faster, hand me your phone now!" She was still screaming. I saw how angry she was, her eyes wide open, and her saliva sprayed in front of me. I was curious about why. She continued screaming and asked me to explain why I talked to someone while they were out. I told her, "Ma'am, I was cleaning the whole day, and someone called me; I didn't see who was calling, and I said hello a few times, but no one answered my call, so I hung up and continued cleaning." She yelled, "You are a liar! Liar, liar, liar!" Then I began to cry; I couldn't stand the way she screamed at me. But I didn't say anything; I just stood there listening and staring at her. She almost slapped my face and told me, "Sir, is going to throw you inside the underground tonight if you don't tell us the truth! Sir, will bury you alive! He will do that! In Saudi Arabia, you are not allowed to lie; you will be killed!"

I was shivering, and I didn't know what I was supposed to do. I couldn't put my mind at ease. In my thoughts, I almost took the knife – I would rather kill myself than be buried alive under their ground. My phone was connected to their internet, or they have access to it, so whenever someone called me, it appeared on their phone. Remember, before they handed me the phone, they had blocked the contact details, so I can't call out, but someone can call my number. Anyway, the number that called me was from a private number, so we couldn't call that number back. I said to the lady employer, "Ma'am, I am so sorry I didn't mean anything. Please forgive me!" I knelt in front of her, and I cried badly. "You have to wait for Sir since you won't tell me the truth!"

After a few hours, I heard someone slam the door. It was the male employer, and he came to the kitchen where I was standing, shivering, and still crying. I said quickly, "Sir, please forgive me, please forgive me!" He was very angry, and I could see that clearly in his face. He used his palm to slam the table. I don't know what I would have done if he had punched me or hurt me that day, but he controlled his emotions. He took paper and pen; then he wrote down what time the caller called me and how many seconds. He spoke to me with an angry voice – a very high and loud voice. He forced me to say something. He wanted me to say what conversation I had with the caller.

He asked me if I gave their address, my name, and other details. I couldn't answer him quickly because I was sobbing, and my throat was already painful. He still continued shouting at me for no reason. I already told them many times the caller didn't say anything. The same as with the lady employer. He was not satisfied with my answer, and he called me a liar. Then he added, "Do you know how dangerous it is to talk to someone else, especially strangers? They can find out where we live, and our lives will be in danger!" Again, I apologized, and finally, I knelt in front of him. Still, he wouldn't forgive me. He took my phone and said, "You will never see this phone again." Before he closed the door, he uttered something in their language. I was so shocked. I couldn't believe what I had heard from the lady and from the male employer. After that day, I couldn't sleep or focus on my work.

Three days later, the lady took me to her parent's house. Both of the couples didn't talk to me at all. I didn't have any idea what was on their minds. I could feel something wasn't right. Mostly because the lady employer told me, "Sir will throw you under our ground, and no one can save your life! You will be buried alive."

Mary noticed that I didn't talk. Then she spoke to me, "I can't call your mobile phone. It says 'the number you had dialed can't be reached at the moment.'" I began to cry and told the helpers everything. I told Mary, "I have been scared ever since the couple mentioned throwing me under the ground." Mary and the rest of the helpers were worried. They advised me to keep praying and be nice to them. Then I told them my plan since I was terrified and needed to do something about the thought of being buried alive. Both of them agreed and pretended that they didn't hear anything from me.

Chapter 44:

Fear of Being Killed

The lady employer picked me up late at night. Again, she didn't talk to me. I just followed her, carrying their daughter's stuff. I cooked dinner as I read notes on their table. I didn't feel like living in that place with those kinds of people around me. It was hurting me badly. I thought about the lady on the plane who said that many helpers had been killed by employers. I couldn't put my mind at ease, no matter how I tried to sleep. I cleaned properly but with no appreciation from the employer. They gave me dirty looks.

While I was typing this, I suddenly remembered how the other man treated me while I was in their house cleaning the kitchen. First, the doctor showed me magazines from Thailand; the magazines were all about underwear. He called my name, "Amanda, look at these magazines." I pretended I didn't hear what he said. He stood up and held the magazines in front of my eyes, showing the lingerie. I was vacuuming at the time, and he was supposed to be sleeping, which was why the wife asked me to clean their house, cook his lunch, and iron his uniform. The doctor followed me around, even as I tried to stay away from him. I had to finish the task given to me. The doctor asked me which pair of underwear I would like so he could buy it for me.

Of course! I sensed quickly he was up to something. I responded to him, "I don't need anything, Sir." I quickly ran into the kitchen, and I closed the door. He knocked on the door, and he said he needed water. I opened the door. While I was washing their dishes, he came to me holding the stethoscope. He said he heard from the wife that I was sick and offered to check on me. He is a Doctor, anyway. First, he said, "The weather is hot, Amanda, you should remove the cover on your head. Don't worry; I mingle with lots of Filipino's in the hospital."

I was curious because, of course, I had been told not to talk to any man, including my employer or family members, and especially always to cover my head. When the doctor spoke, I didn't respond to him. He came close to me, he said one more time, "Amanda, I'll check on you. Don't worry; there isn't anybody here. Ma'am is out, and she'll be back only in the evening." He grabbed the cover off my hair and forcefully dropped it to the floor. I continued to wash the dishes, and he kept talking to me. I faced him, and I said, "Sir, I'm sorry, but I am not allowed to talk to any men or else I'll get into big trouble. I am already taking my medicines." Then he said, "Amanda, let me check on you to make sure you are okay."

Since it seemed he had a good intention, I was forced to sit, and he checked on my back; then, suddenly, he asked me to remove my uniform so he can check on my breast. I refused and quickly stood up. I told him, "Sir, I have lots of work to do, and don't scare me." I saw him shivering like he wanted to do something at that moment. Even If I shouted, nobody could hear me. Thank God! He went into his room and closed their door. I was nervous and scared. He did this to me many times, he tried to commit something, but I always made a way to escape. I couldn't tell my employers this since they are already hated me and were still not talking to me at all.

When I was done with my chores, I went down to my employer's house. There I saw a note and a Nokia phone. I read the note, and it said, "You can use this phone for our child's purposes."

During the night time, my rest time, I still couldn't put my mind at ease. My mind was dictating to me - I checked on the phone to see whether I could use it to call in the Philippines. I sent a short message to my family. "I can't really stand to stay any longer in this house. It has been months already. They didn't take me to see Mary, Susanne, and Laila."

After a few minutes, my family called back. I told them I couldn't talk much because I was facing a huge problem. My family was curious and nervous. I told them I'd explain once it was settled and asked them to cooperate with me at that time. I deleted the message I had sent to my family from the sent folder. I made sure they can't trace any calls or messages. It so happens both of the couples were busy working, and the wife was busy studying. That week was her exam, so she needed to focus on her studies. Then they brought me to the other house to do general cleaning because they were expecting guests the next day. I went there while their daughter stayed in the other house.

I had just started cleaning when I saw the man wrapped with a towel on his lower body. I tried to avoid him. I slowly closed the door and start cleaning their second floor instead of cleaning the first floor first. He was there, so how could I clean and focus. He kept walking towards me until he spoke to me. "Hi Amanda, how are you? You seem tired. How's your family? Would you mind changing our bed sheet first?" He went out and watched television. He was sitting and eating, so I quickly went to their room because I respect the wife, who asked me to clean their house even if the husband was around. I was almost done changing their bedsheet.

When I was almost finished, the doctor was behind me, and he quickly hugged me very tightly. I couldn't move, I couldn't shout. He was naked! I saw everything! I begged him not to do anything. Then, he begged me to massage his private parts so he won't do any harm to me. "I am facing a problem already. Please don't add some more, Sir." I pushed him hard, but I really couldn't move. I used all my strength to escape from him. He held me tightly. He was very strong! I was hurting. He is tall and big. He warned me, "I want you to massage my private parts, or else you will be in a dangerous situation."

I didn't finish cleaning their house. I couldn't concentrate. I went back to my employer's home. There I waited for my employer to come back from university. I prepared myself for my own benefits and safety so I can save my life from this horrible place. I used my family's text messages as evidence. After a few hours, the lady came back. The moment she entered the door, I quickly ran to her, crying terribly, hugged her, and said, "Ma'am, my husband died due to a car accident. He just died; my family just called me. Ma'am and they texted me." I showed her my phone. I was really crying. For the first time, I heard her voice again, talking to me.

I was still crying, pretended to be in shock, and pretended that I don't know what I was doing. Then the lady called the husband. I was in the kitchen the whole time, didn't eat, still in my dirty and wet uniform. It was already night time when the male employer came back home. He quickly entered the kitchen and said, "I'm sorry for your loss. I will book your plane ticket tonight so you can go back home within two days." The next day, the lady employer took me to Mary's place. The moment I went down from their car, I saw Laila, Marivic, and Mary cleaning the wide garage. They stared at me hard. They hated what I had done. Mary's eyes rolled and looked at me sharply, and I could see in her actions how mad she was. I was hurt, and none of them understood what I went through with my employer. I begged them not to say anything, or else all of us would be in trouble. They didn't talk to me either until the lady employer picked me up.

I packed my things, but I didn't take all my things as I am allowed only to take a few clothes since they expect me to come back. The male employer told me, your plane ticket is already booked, and the ticket was expensive. Then the lady employer came, she gave me a necklace as her gift. The next day around 9:00 a.m., I was waiting in the kitchen, crying and sobbing. Once again, they checked my things before leaving their house. I secretly left a letter in the kitchen. I wrote something great about them. I was appreciating how amazing they were and that I was grateful for everything they had done for me starting from the first day.

We went out of their big house, and the couple dropped me off at the airport. I was quiet while we were on our way. I remember how nice they treat me during that day. Deep inside, I wasn't happy that I lied. However, I am happy because I was finally about to escape from that scary place.

Chapter 45:
Trouble at the
Saudi Arabia Airport

The male employer accompanied me all the way inside the airport. I felt bad because he was so nice that day. I felt guilty, but I knew I had to save my life before something happened to me. I carried just two bags since I was allowed to carry only 20 kg. After one hour, the male employer had to leave since he needed to go to work. He said goodbye to me, waving his hand with pity on his face. He felt bad about me because he believed that my husband died. I knew this wasn't the right thing to do, but it was done.

The couple was already gone from the airport. During the weighing of luggage, I found I had exceeded my weight allowance. The guy who was in charge of weighing luggage at the airport said. "I'm sorry you can't carry all these items. You have to remove some because your employer only booked 20kg." I didn't know what to do at that time; they told me to call my employer to settle or else just go to the trash bin and throw away the excess items. I told the guy that my employer already left. I begged them many times because I have only a little money. If I spent my little money, I'd be empty-handed. I still needed to take the bus once I reached Manila. I kept crying and crying - the plane had only 20 minutes left before it left. The guy ignored me and left me to think of a way to pay for the excess baggage.

I kept sobbing in a corner; I begged everyone to let me go in since I had just 10 minutes left. But all of them said that they were sorry and were just following the rules and regulations. "You can call your employer and let them pick you up and rebook your ticket." That was painful to hear. I told myself the items inside were important, but if that was the case, then I didn't have a choice anymore. Then suddenly, a young Saudi guy asks me to go in with my luggage. I was so happy that he saved me. Can you imagine being in a terrible mess and it working out at the last moment? If you could see how I looked then like I just escaped from a mental hospital. I was helpless.

I went quickly on the plane, and 10 minutes later, the plane's engine started. What a good feeling, I whispered to myself. I was stressed and still worried. I was praying hard that I could reach the Philippines before they found out I lied because they could call immigration and stop me from flying back home. It was a long trip, and I kept quiet on the plane. I didn't talk to anyone and kept to myself because I was afraid to share my secret. When I left Saudi Arabia, it was wintertime. It was cold; my hands and fingers were fully cracked – anyone would notice that I was a hardworking person.

My journey to Saudi Arabia was mysterious. I experienced many trials and pains, and I struggled a lot. There were many sleepless nights. I couldn't stand any longer how those people treated me, expecting me to work non-stop. Thank God! I saved my own life. I knew the three helpers wouldn't be affected since we didn't care much for each other. Of course, they won't be hurt because of my actions. I learned only how to save my own life. However, I am grateful that they cooperated with me.

Yes! Finally, Emirates Airlines was about to land at the Philippines Airport. I could feel the smile on my face. I was happy, but I was thinking about going to the hospital first. The moment I came down from the plane, I went to the hospital to book an appointment for them to operate on me without spending too much money. I suffered from terrible headaches for more than three years. I ignored my health before, and even though my employer knew about my situation, they didn't care much. I wasn't going to ignore my health any longer.

I remember it was exactly 4:00 a.m. when I was queued at the hospital to get a slot. So many people were queuing. If I wasn't mistaken, I was number 119. When I met the doctor, he said the cysts were big and grew close to my nostrils. He also found out that my thyroid was enlarged, and he checked on it to make sure I didn't have a goiter. He didn't find anything suspicious. The doctor told me there was nothing to worry about there. But he told me both of my nostrils were infected. He checked on my nostrils through screening machines (I forget what they call that machine) saw that the big cysts that grew close to my nostrils were making it hard for me to breathe well and could be causing my migraine and blurred eyesight. I didn't go back to my hometown yet because I need to stay in Manila for a couple of days. I was grateful because the doctor asked me to buy only a few things for the surgery, and the surgery was free. He asked me to buy a surgical mask, surgical head cover, and surgical aprons. It costs me only P150. The doctor told me to come back after three days. I called my family and let them know I'd be in the hospital. I told them I missed them so badly, and I wanted to see them, but I had to settle my health first. I knew my family needed the money since I hadn't sent any money that month.

While waiting for the day of my surgery, I stayed in Manila. You can't live without money in the city. It's tough; you have to buy everything, including water. I starved myself since I wanted to save money. After three days, I went early to the hospital, carrying all the stuff. I submitted all of my documents to the counter and waited five hours for my name to be called.

I was still wearing the necklace my employer gave to me. It was cute, 21k with a heart pendant. I heard my name called from the operating room. I removed my necklace and quickly threw it inside my bag. I was nervous and tried to breathe. Inhale, exhale, inhale, exhale. It was my first time having to undergo such surgery. I was 28 years old. The doctors asked me to lie down, then sprayed anesthesia into both of my nostrils. After 10 minutes, they started the surgery. The assistant nurse held my hands tightly while the doctor started to pull out the cysts little by little. I could feel the pain even though they used anesthesia. I saw the small jar or bottle that they used to keep whatever flesh had been removed. About eleven times, they pulled pieces out of my nose. I could feel the tears drop on my cheek. "Can you please add more anesthesia? I can still feel the pain." The doctor said there would only be a few more seconds before it was finished.

After the surgery, I felt weak and giddy. Then the doctor pulled out a long cotton strip and inserted it inside my nose to prevent bleeding. I don't know exactly know how they could call that cotton. Then the doctor asked me to come back after 14 days to remove the cotton. It was already irritating me so badly, blocking one nostril. I bought my medicines and still stayed in Manila. I had to settle everything before going back home to my hometown. I quickly checked that the necklace was still in my bag, but I found out it was missing. I removed everything looking for it. I told myself, this might be my karma for lying. I went out of the hospital with plasters on my nose, walking by myself. While I was walking, I talked to my own shadow. I could get over it - this is the first and the last surgery I ever had in my life.

While I was lying down, I received a call. I couldn't identify the caller because the number didn't appear. When I answered it, I heard the lady's employer voice over the line. I was wondering who gave my number to her. Then I remember I called Marivic, which means she gave my number to the lady employer. She was talking non-stop. She cursed me and said, "Amanda, you are a liar; you lied to us! Starting today onwards, you and your family will suffer. One of your family members will die, and we are going to pray to Allah. Do you know how powerful and strong our prayer is? You will suffer till the end of your life. No matter what you do, you will never ever become successful. You said your husband died from a car accident? Liar, liar, liar, I hate you, Amanda!"

I told her, "Please forgive me for not telling you the truth. You and Sir scared me so badly by threatening me. You remember Ma'am, you said, Sir, can throw me under the ground alive? Ma'am, do you think that sounds good? Did you know the moment I heard that I slashed my pulse and almost killed myself? Did you remember when I was rushed to the hospital? I purposely hurt myself, slashed my own wrist because I was scared. It is not my fault that I made way for me to be able to escape from that scary place."

I added, "One more thing, I was almost raped by your brother-in-law. I didn't need to wait for something to happen to me before I take action. I am sorry, and please forgive me." The lady responded, "I will never ever forgive you, Amanda. You will pay for it. The plane ticket is very expensive, and you have to pay for it."

She hung up the phone, and she sent me messages that were extremely hurtful. I messaged her back to ask for forgiveness, and I told her, "Ma'am, you have to remember, I was a servant for more than three years with two families. Before I said yes to Mary, she only mentioned one family. I didn't complain about that. I slept only three hours almost every day - you didn't hear any complaints from me. So please, Ma'am, don't ask me to pay for

the plane ticket. I did my best. Please forgive me."
She replied back with more hurtful words.

Laila's mom called me. "Amanda, we are now
scared that they might hurt our daughter in Saudi
Arabia. We want her to come back to the
Philippines as soon as possible." Everybody blamed
me. Since then, I have changed my number so
nobody could contact me. I turned off my phone. I
wanted to have peace of mind. I just got out of the
hospital, and my body needed lots of rest.

Fourteen days seemed way too long for me to wait.
The doctor said I have to go back to the hospital to
remove the cotton he inserted in my nose, but I
couldn't wait any longer. I had very little money left
in my wallet. I couldn't survive if I continued to
stay. I needed to pay for the room rent and buy
food since I couldn't cook where I was staying. I
called the hospital to arrange an earlier
appointment. They agreed.

The next day I went to the hospital, queued many
hours as I went down late in the morning. When I
met the doctor, he said, "you should wait for
exactly fourteen days." I told the doctor, "I have to

go overseas in the next three days, and I need to go back to my hometown first." The doctor pulled the cotton slowly. I saw lots of thick blood drops on my white t-shirt. Then the doctor quickly took more cotton and inserted it in my nose. "This was the reason we couldn't pull out the cotton; the scars haven't healed. That's why you are bleeding," the doctor added.

The doctor said he wanted to see me after two years because both of my nostrils got affected. This means there are also small cysts that grew inside the other nostril. I thanked the doctor and went out of the hospital with the bloodstains on my shirt. I packed my things and went back to my hometown. As I walked, I saw everybody staring at me because of the bandages on my nose. They probably thought I got a nose job!

It was raining when I went down from the bus. I walked through the muddy, rainy, and rough rocky road of the hillside. I was so excited to see my family. I bought fish and doughnuts for the kids. After 25 minutes of walking, finally, I had reached my parent's house. There I saw my kids, sisters, nieces, and parents busy harvesting charcoals.

Poor people! When I left them, they were busy making charcoal, and this time was the same.

Chapter 46:
The Art of Giving

Our house was still the same. I didn't have a chance to improve anything this time. I was alone supporting my family. It has been tough, but I have to be strong.

You might be wondering about my husband. I have to be honest here. He doesn't have a stable job as he is suffering from illnesses. I am stressed. However, I didn't allow my family to see that. I didn't want them to pity me. I wanted to rest and sleep, but seeing my family members like this still, I couldn't rest. My daughters were so dirty, with runny noses and long, dirty nails. Sigh! What a pity. I unpacked my luggage and took out a few snacks for the kids.

No matter how tired I was, I managed to teach the kids to wash their hands before picking up or touching any snacks to prevent sickness. Yes, I grew up in the mountains, but I learned the value of cleanliness at 13 when I first started working as a helper.

After a few minutes, many visitors came to our house, including our neighbors. As usual, we had to feed people. You can't say to people, "Hi, we are having lunch. Kindly come back later." That's rude, right? We were always very hospitable to guests. The visitors stayed until late at night. This was a reality. They couldn't go back to their houses empty-handed. You should share with them at least soaps, toothpaste from overseas, clothes, dried goods, or anything. This is how we lived in the Philippines.

Our life on the hillside consisted of almost the same activity or cycle every single day. Nothing much changed after I worked so hard overseas. Our house is still the same, and I didn't have any savings. The only investment I had for three years, eight months of working overseas was the land I bought close to the city. I was beginning to realize that working alone wasn't that easy. I couldn't blame my family either since our mindset is so different. I love to explore new things and get out of my comfort zone while my family wants to stick to what they have always done, believing 'this is the life we are destined to live.' I stayed in my parent's house while thinking about how to apply for a job in another country. I thought of submitting my resume to different agencies in Manila since I finished a degree course.

I wanted to work in a hotel. I am okay with any job, but my dream when I was in secondary school was to work at the front desk in a hotel. The problem was that I didn't have experience working in a hotel except for housekeeping. Deep inside my heart, even though I didn't have experience with that kind of industry, I knew that I could do a good job. After all, I started working as a maid for different rich families. However, the hotel managers were looking for those who underwent a training course, graduated with the same category degree, and had at least two years of experience working at a hotel.

I was bored staying in our place. I couldn't buy my own necessities, not even shampoo. I felt sorry for my kids having to eat unhealthy foods because we didn't have any vegetables to harvest. We needed to wait at least four months before the plants would produce vegetables.

I hated seeing my family suffer. You might be wondering why I allowed myself to starve like that if there's a lot of food in the mountain. I get what you are thinking, and I used to think the same way, too. There are many ways to find food, but there are times when everything you need can't be found. We were lucky if, during rainy days, there were mushrooms growing. I went out and checked all of the banana trees, and there I harvested many organic mushrooms. We enjoyed having simple food.

I would go out to harvest green papayas from very far places, then carry them all the way home. Then my mom was the one who sold the papaya to the market. Sometimes my mom would give away the papaya since too many other people were selling papayas in the market. Mostly she bought milk for my kids. She loved her granddaughters so much.

Through incidents in my life, I have always realized that the power of giving is divine. It changes not only the giver but also the receiver. Giving and receiving is an art. When someone gives you something, you must learn how to receive it. Never take a giver for granted. Remember that a giver is a messenger of the Universe. When the Universe is giving you through someone, you must acknowledge, respect, and accept the gift with all your heart and soul.

---------- *END OF VOLUME I* ----------

THANK YOU

VOLUME I – Amanda Nav wants to sincerely thank you for choosing to read Volume I of Amanda Nav's **From Helper to Fitness Coach**. It is all about the journey. This book shows how life can treat you when you let things happen without understanding yourself and choosing the right goals. Most of the time, you will find your life spiraling out of control. With faith and a little self-confidence, you can create harmony, but you will be lost in the noise of this world.

VOLUME II – This part will show you how Amanda worked on the roots, which is the mindset, and took control of her life. She started designing her own life in the ways she wanted. She stopped being the victim of the situation and started demanding from the Universe with grace and laser-like focus. Do pre-order this copy as this will transform your life FOREVER!!!

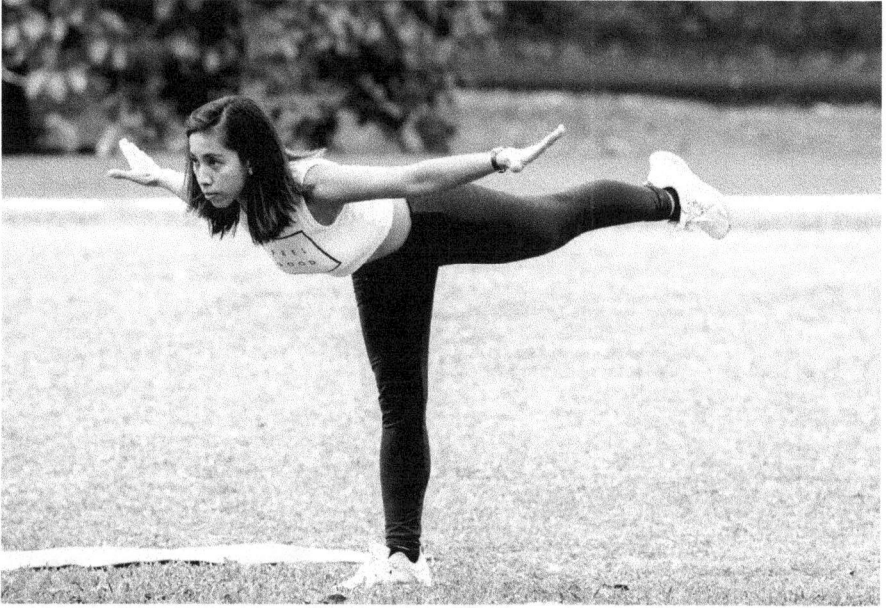

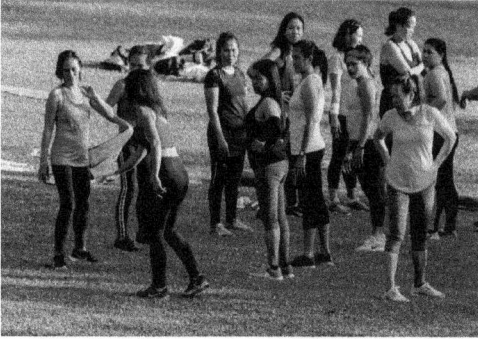
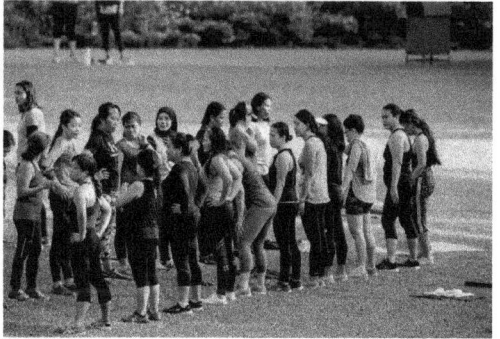

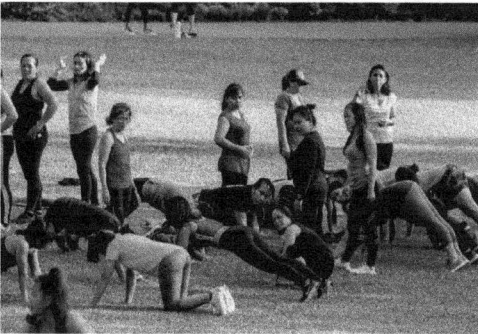
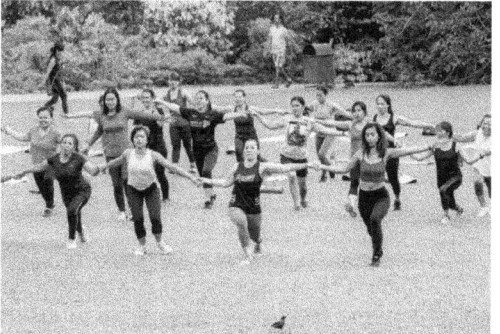

www.ingramcontent.com/pod-product-compliance
Lightning Source LLC
Chambersburg PA
CBHW060447280326
41933CB00014B/2694